M000206576

Restless Leg Syndrome RLS

From A Restless Leg Sufferer To A Restless Leg Sufferer

How I solved my RLS with a bag of sand!

With 83 Home Remedies.

by

Emily Eldeston

ALL RIGHTS RESERVED. This book contains material protected under International and Federal Copyright Laws and Treaties.

Any unauthorized reprint or use of this material is strictly prohibited. No part of this book may be reproduced or transmitted in any form or by any means, electronic, mechanical or otherwise, including photocopying or recording, or by any information storage and retrieval system without express written permission from the author.

Copyrighted © 2015

Published by: IMB Publishing

Table of Contents

Table of Contents

Table of Contents

Introduction

I have been a Restless Leg Syndrome (RLS) sufferer for over 10 years. I just couldn't get to sleep at night. On a typical night, I would toss and turn, get up, walk around, put some cream on, try to get to sleep again, get up again; until I eventually fell asleep at 4 or 5 am knowing I have to get up 4 hours later.

I told my husband that I would make it a priority to solve my RLS so I started practicing EVERYTHING I could find that could possibly help me without medication. The doctors don't know what causes my RLS and want to give me tablets but I refuse to take them as I hate taking medication.

Endless visits to the doctors and all possible treatments did not help me get rid of this annoying feeling in my legs that seemed to creep up any time I would lay down. All the insomnia and also the phobia of socialising, due to lack of sleep, led to mounting frustration with nowhere to vent it out.

The biggest relief came when I realised that I was not alone, when I was starting to research my symptoms. There are several people who suffer from a similar condition. I found out many names for this condition. People called it "shift legs", "itchy bones" and several other things. I did not know what problem I had. I did not even know that this is a medically recognised condition. All I knew was that it made my life miserable. I was perpetually exhausted and irritable. It was only when I was introduced to another person with the same condition that I found some solace. A million thanks to my friend who made this meeting possible.

That is when I was introduced to the condition. I was told that the condition is called "Restless Leg Syndrome". It is strange how the mind works sometimes. I was so happy to know what problem I have. If it was recognised as a disorder, there must be some cure for it as well. If it is medically recognised, then I most definitely had hope. This is when my search for the ultimate cure for Restless Leg Syndrome or RLS began. In the process, I realised that there is so much more to this condition than just the cure.

I also spoke to many people who suffered from worse than just sleepless nights. One such story was of a lady whose entire family was distraught because of her condition. She was under medication to fall asleep. However, there was absolutely no relief from the constant movement of her legs. She would be up all night, walking around the house and just keeping her restless feet occupied. The condition worsened to a level where she would actually fall asleep in the bathtub with water jets directed at the feet. Imagine being in and out of the tub each night. As sadistic as this may sound, I felt comfort to know that I was not that bad yet.

Because of these troubled nights, my friend was always irritable. She was unable to maintain relationships and this led to a broken marriage. The trauma that she experienced led to finding ways to stay relaxed. Lucky for her, she was able to find some solution to her restlessness in the form of dopamine medication. But when she was off the medication, the walking around and experiencing the creepiest feeling in the legs resumed.

Another person I spoke to was able to sleep in just one position all night to prevent the restlessness in her legs. While this solved RLS, it led to problems like persistent back pain. She went to several doctors who were unable to figure out why she was always complaining of pain and restlessness despite being able to sleep. It wasn't until a neurologist took her blood samples that she realised that she had Restless Leg Syndrome. It was only after that that her symptoms were managed better. She was able to calm her "shifty legs" and was able to switch positions during sleep.

These are just two stories of the hundreds of people that I have spoken to and read about. Some stories are really heart breaking. It is unsettling to know that people suffer with sleep deprivation for a large part of their adult lives. The worst part is that they do not even know why. Quite similar to my story, I guess. For so many years, I did not even know that my condition even had a name. There is such little information available about RLS that it is quite natural for people to be clueless about this condition.

Many relate RLS to other conditions like Diabetes. Others believe that a long standing back injury is the cause for the restlessness in their legs. The common thread that I have found in all this stories is that at some point everyone reaches a state of hopelessness. You begin to believe that you are destined to be unable to get rest or even socialise without the prospect of embarrassing spasms.

I am determined to help people out of this misery. That is why I spoke to several doctors and even people suffering from this condition. I have gathered a lot of information about Restless Leg Syndrome that has helped me find some comfort over the last couple of years. There are several remedies that people have tried. Some of them worked for me, some didn't. Nevertheless, I will share it all with you, hoping that you will find relief from the most annoying condition that is Restless Leg Syndrome.

I expect this book to be a one stop solution to all your questions about RLS. I also urge you to visit forums and talk to people about the condition. There is always a lot to explore about this rather interesting and less studied condition.

My RLS only ever starts when I lay down e.g. watching TV or when I go to sleep so I never have RLS sitting down.

Chapter 1: Getting to Know the Condition

The most important thing to do when you are suffering from any condition is to understand how it affects the body. The communication that is occurring within your body is responsible for making it react in a certain way. That is what doctors call pathophysiology.

Now, Restless Leg Syndrome can occur on its own. That is when there is no other condition along with Restless Leg Syndrome. That is when the condition is known as Primary Restless Leg Syndrome. Now, if the condition is caused by some other problem such as the deficiency of certain nutrients, it is called Secondary Restless Leg Syndrome. The changes that occur in the body vary as per the type of RLS you are experiencing. We will discuss this in a little more detail in the following sections of the chapter. In this book, I will, most often, refer to the condition, simply as RLS, Restless Leg Syndrome, as I don't know if your RLS is Primary or Secondary.

1. Common Symptoms of Restless Leg Syndrome

The next thing to worry about is understanding the symptoms of RLS. The sad thing is that many people never know for a long time what the condition actually is. Here are some common statements that I have heard from people who have the condition but do not know what it really is:

"I can feel burning sensations at the tip of my feet"

"My toes feel weird"

"I can feel very unpleasant sensations that go away when I shake my legs around"

"My legs just feel horrible all the time, like ants crawling all over my legs"

All these signs appear in the initial period of Restless Leg Syndrome. The symptoms may get severe and can also lead to extreme pain and discomfort; this why Restless Leg Syndrome is often confused with several other neurological conditions. It is important for you to recognise the symptoms at the earliest so that you can seek treatment when the condition is still moderate.

Some sufferers never have twitching legs but just the creepy, crawly feeling as soon as they lay down for longer than 5 minutes. I belong in this category. I don't have uncontrollable twitching legs at all. Having said that, I do want to move and shake my legs to try and make my legs feel better but these movements are controlled by me.

Below are symptoms that are most common for Restless Leg Syndrome:

An urge to move your legs

This is one of the first symptoms required to diagnose your condition as Restless leg Syndrome. When I began to experience it in the beginning, it was actually quite scary. There used to be strange sensations in my legs that would go away only when I shook my legs really hard. If you are also feeling these uncomfortable sensations, just when you are about to fall asleep, you possibly have RLS.

For me, these sensations would occur every night so I knew that it would be a long and tiring night, again. The intensity of these symptoms varies greatly. For some it is just a quick jerk that can ease the sensations and for others violent movements of the leg also fail to ease the unusual and unpleasant feeling in the legs.

If you talk to anyone with Restless Leg Syndrome, they would describe the sensations as tugging, itching, pulling, burning, prickling, tingling, jittery, "creepy crawly" and gnawing feelings.

These itchy sensations are not on the skin or the surface. It seems like they reach right down to your bones. For others, the feeling is similar to a hundred creepy crawly insects or worms moving up and down their legs.

Some sufferers have uncontrollable movements of their legs: these jerky movements start off as voluntary movements and can end up being repetitive and involuntary. When the movements become violent and uncontrollable, you need to be prepared for sleepless nights. You cannot sleep through these movements. They may also turn into severe cramps in the calf region. The pain throbs throughout the entire leg and can leave tingling sensations even when the pain is gone.

Inability to remain asleep

The problem with these movements is that they occur periodically. For this reason, they are also known as Periodic Limb Movements. Sometimes, they can occur every 30 second, making it impossible for you to fall asleep. They may be persistent for a few minutes and then recur in intervals throughout the night.

Naturally, it makes it impossible for a person to fall asleep. This is the most common problem with anyone who has been diagnosed with Restless Leg Syndrome, although not all people have Periodic Limb Movements.

This symptom is not necessary for you to be diagnosed with Restless Leg Syndrome. However, it is one of the most common complaints among individuals with this problem. If you are up, reading books, watching TV or just trying to get some relief from the painful sensations in your leg, it may help you to know that you are not alone. This is a supportive symptom for the diagnosis of this condition. You must make sure you discuss it with your doctor when you go for treatment.

The problem is that many individuals believe that sleeplessness is an obvious result of Restless Leg Syndrome. However, it could also be your sleep pattern which is the cause for your Restless Leg Syndrome. Sometimes, we are unable to fall asleep due to several reasons like stress and emotional distress. These issues may manifest themselves in the form of extremely uncontrollable neurological sensations that are painful.

Movement eases the symptoms

This is a very important criterion for diagnosis. In my case, I used to get immediate relief from the tingling sensations when I started to walk around the house. Even wiggling my legs used to work sometimes. I was told that this relief when you move the limbs is the most sure shot symptom of Restless Leg Syndrome. But one can't walk around all night, so I had to find another remedy, which I will talk about later.

For many people who are suffering from this condition, the relief is only temporary. But, they do feel the relief, nevertheless. For other lucky ones, the relief is complete as soon as some activity or movement starts. They feel completely relieved from these sensations until the movement continues. Once it stops, the pain is back.

However, the goal is to get some relief from the pain/sensation. So, people tend to move around and walk around irrespective of the fact that they are unable to get any sleep.

The symptoms become worse when you are resting

No matter what type of sensation you are feeling, whether it is a tingling feeling in your toes or cramps, they get worse when you are at rest. The moment you stop moving or decide to retire for the day, your symptoms just become uncontrollable. Especially when you are lying down, you have uncomfortable and unpleasant feelings in your legs. This increase in the symptoms towards the evening is important for diagnosis. Like I mentioned before, symptoms of Restless Leg Syndrome are cyclic. They tend to follow a pattern that needs to be understood for diagnosis.

Most often, the pattern repeats itself at night and becomes severe with time.

Night time Twitching

For some people RLS symptoms occur along with Periodic Leg movements. This appears in the form of sudden jerking or twitching of the legs while you are asleep. These movements can disrupt sleep to a large extent, making it difficult for you to get any rest.

2. Daytime Symptoms

For most people, the symptoms of Restless Leg Syndrome aggravate in the evenings. The real problem occurs when you start experiencing these problems during the day. Sometimes, when you are just sitting down and relaxing, the unpleasant sensations along with violent jerking of the leg might occur during the day. The basic thing is that whenever your legs are at rest, they feel unpleasant. Usually, moving around will solve the issue during the day. When you divert your attention from these unpleasant sensations, you might get relief from the symptoms almost immediately.

However, there are other things you need to worry about if you are experiencing these symptoms during the day. If you are driving and are stuck in a traffic jam, it is possible for you to have creepy feelings and even pain in your leg. Involuntary movements in the legs may also occur in your legs, making it difficult or dangerous for you to drive.

I personally have not met anyone who has experienced this problem when they are driving. I have only read blogs and forums. However, I do know that several people who suffer from this condition tend to have aggravated symptoms when they are sitting in the passenger's seat. This is when the legs are at rest. So the symptoms may occur.

The next thing you need to worry about is workplace hazards. You may have accidents at your workplace if restlessness occurs elsewhere other than your legs. We will talk about symptoms in other body parts in the next section. Another problem is sleeplessness which can also lead to unwanted accidents if you are handling machinery or heavy equipment. So, make sure you speak to your doctor in detail about your profession when you are seeking any sort of assistance or treatment.

If you have experienced RLS symptoms during the day, it is a good idea to make sure that you are moving around regularly. Even if you have a job that confines you to a desk or a cabin all day, make sure you move your legs around to prevent symptoms. In case you do experience these symptoms suddenly, you can just take a walk around your office to feel relieved. I know many people who constantly move their ankles or rotate them to ensure that the symptoms do not occur during the day.

Psychological effects of Restless Leg Syndrome during the day cannot be ignored. You may feel embarrassed to take the subway or even sit in a restaurant because you are unable to predict when the symptoms may manifest. You may also notice that your performance at work also falls short considerably.

Remember that you are not alone in this. There are several people who are dealing with far worse symptoms during the day. All you need to make sure is that you keep your legs active. If the symptoms are in any other body part, you can try simple movements and exercises to prevent the symptoms during the day.

3. Symptoms in Other Body Parts

Similar symptoms of RLS are experienced in other parts of the body as well. The sensations are the same as you would feel in the legs. For most people, the symptoms occur in the region between the knee and the ankle. If you pay some attention to the symptoms that occur in the other parts of the body, you might be able to control RLS from becoming more intense. The symptoms occur mostly in the thighs, the back and the arms besides the legs.

Symptoms in the arms: Sometimes, people experience tingling sensations in their arms. These sensations begin during the onset of RLS. The sensations are very similar to the ones you feel in your leg. It is creepy, painful and feels like someone is pinching your entire arm. The sensations come and go. It repeats every 30 seconds and can get worse at nights.

Many times, these symptoms go unrecognised. You see, the name Restless Leg Syndrome can be misleading. We expect the symptoms to occur only in the legs. However, when you begin to feel these sensations, you must observe them. If they are cyclic, get better when you move the limb around and also occur when your arm is resting, then it is most probably RLS.

You may also experience numbness suddenly. If you can verify the other three conditions mentioned above, even numbness is considered to be the initial phase of Restless Leg Syndrome. When you are able to understand these symptoms, you can prevent them from spreading to your legs and other body parts.

Symptoms in the back: Restless Leg Syndrome is often a neurological condition. This means that your spine is at the core of the condition. So, it is not abnormal to experience these symptoms in your back. Most often, the symptoms are experienced in your lower back. There may not be any violent jerks as such. However, you can experience cringing pain and tingling sensations in your back. This may occur at the onset or can also spread from your legs to your back. Either way, when the problem is in the back, you must pay attention to it.

With the back, movement to ease the symptoms is a difficult option. Of course, when you are able to stretch or move around, the symptoms will reduce. When you lie down, the symptoms aggravate. Even when you are sitting or watching television, you may feel the painful sensations.

Besides the back and the arms, you may feel the symptoms of RLS in your thighs as well. For some really unfortunate people, the symptoms occur all over the body. The options to reduce the symptoms when they are so severe are available. However you need to be more consistent with the treatment. You may also have to make drastic lifestyle changes to feel free from the symptoms.

4. RLS Symptoms in Children and Infants

The real difficulty in diagnosing symptoms of Restless Leg Syndrome comes with infants and children. It is not an uncommon condition among children. In the USA alone, close to 1.5 million children are affected with Restless Leg Syndrome. For most adults suffering from the condition, the onset is during childhood. Most people I know have ignored the symptoms in their childhood. So what started off as a mild or moderate symptom went on to becoming a lot more severe.

I was intrigued by this early onset of the symptoms and decided to do some research on why this condition goes unnoticed in infants. The statistics that I came across were shocking enough to motivate this research. Did you know that in almost 35% of the adults who have been diagnosed with Restless Leg Syndrome, the symptoms manifest when they are children or infants?

It is most difficult when the condition is seen in infants. The first thing that most parents notice is that the baby does not fall asleep easily. Even when the child sleeps, it seems to be disturbed. But, this is a condition that you will observe even in babies who do not have RLS. Now, this is what makes it so hard to point out the condition as RLS.

As for the movement of the legs, we all know that babies tend to move their limbs around in order to keep themselves entertained. This is a form of play that most infants indulge in. So, when there are jerks or sudden movements in the legs, parents tend to ignore them as an intentional movement.

The other problem is that the infant is unable to describe the sensations. They are unable to point out to the tingling or painful sensations. You will notice that the baby is irritable. Sleep is definitely an issue. In addition to that, they are also unable to eat well. They tend to cry all day long because of Restless Leg Syndrome. They are mostly likened to other childhood disorders as the symptoms go undetected.

In slightly older children, the symptoms could be mild or severe. Irrespective of the intensity of the symptoms, the impact it has on the quality of the child's life is negative. Just like adults, children realise that they can get some relief from the symptoms of Restless Leg Syndrome by moving around. You will notice that they tend to rock constantly, change positions often when they are in bed, run really fast, stretch and even walk around the house.

In case of children, the symptoms may also occur during the day. They tend to show the same type of movement in their classroom set up as well. The problem with this is that it is normally likened to inattentiveness and hyperactivity. For this reason, the condition is mostly likened to a psychological disorder. When the child behaves abnormally, parents usually ignore the possibility of associated issues like sleeplessness and irritability. A neurological condition is not even considered a possibility when a child begins to behave differently.

Because of sleeplessness and pain, children tend to exhibit offensive behaviour like anger and disobedience. Children could also be extremely disruptive. The movement of the limbs constantly in class can also be considered a behavioural problem. All these manifestations of Restless Leg Syndrome are also similar to the symptoms of Attention Deficit Hyperactive Disorder. Therefore, even before considering other possibilities, children are treated for ADHD. I also know of parents who feel extremely hopeless because the child does not respond positively to this treatment.

If there is a child or toddler in your house who may be showing the above symptoms, there are four important steps that you need to follow in order to ensure that you are able to provide the right support to help the child cope with the condition:

- Try to understand the cause for discomfort and irritability in the child. This is necessary to continue with any type of treatment.

- Once you know the cause, it is necessary to provide early and timely treatment. You are not only able to eliminate the symptoms but can also prevent them from extending into adulthood.

- You must explore the possible treatment options. There are several medical options and also simple home remedies that can reduce the symptoms in the child.

- Address the sleep disorders first to make sure that the emotional and intellectual issues are sorted.

There are several paediatric patients who complain of Restless Leg Syndrome. This rise in numbers has led to a lot of research about Restless Leg Syndrome in Children and Adolescents. While the symptoms remain the same, there is a huge difference in the diagnosis of the condition in the younger patients.

Another thing you need to understand is the display of these symptoms in children is very different. They will also describe the condition differently. Most often, they will tell you that they can feel spiders, ants or bugs on their legs. They may also refer to them as "oowies". The child may tell you that he has so much energy in his legs that he wants to run. These descriptions may seem vague to an adult who is unaware of Restless Leg Syndrome. However, if you can identify the condition and at least assume the chances that your child has this problem, you will be able to improve the quality of your child's life greatly.

For other children, the leg sensations are not such an important symptom as sleep deprivation. Studies show that by the time a child has reached the age of 11, it is chronic sleep deprivation that precedes all the leg sensations. In these situations, you must consider RLS as a possible or probable condition among several other issues that are causing sleep deprivation. Especially if one of the parents or any family member suffers from Restless Leg Syndrome, you must never rule out or ignore this condition. If the condition is not confirmed or does not have a definite diagnosis, you can move on the other causal factors.

The next part deals with the diagnosis of the condition. There are several stages at which RLS occurs and each one has its own diagnosis.

Chapter 2: Pathophysiology of RLS

With all the research that I have done, I have found that the exact mechanism of RLS is still quite unexplored. There are several theories about this condition. One such theory affiliates the condition to the neurotransmitter dopamine. This is one of the most convincing options available as dopamine treatment has been observed to be quite effective with Restless Leg Syndrome.

With the Dopamine Theory, there is also a connection drawn between another condition called Periodic Limb Movement Disorder. Of course, the pathophysiology is not identical. But, since these conditions tend to occur together most of the times and also because the type of medication provided is also quite similar, it has been assumed that they may also share some similarities in the mechanism. Like all the other proposed mechanisms of RLS, even this one has not been completely proved right.

Several electrophysiological methods have been used to demonstrate that the spinal mechanism in both the conditions is common. There were also several experiments conducted on patients with RLS and also a planned control group. These experiments revealed that the spinal cord was more excitable in patients with RLS. The spatial spread of this excitability and also the low threshold to any stimuli was also more at nights. This data provides enough proof that Periodic Limb Movement Disorder and RLS share one thing in common, which is the excitability of the spinal cord. Similarly, RLS has been associated with several conditions such as myelopathy, peripheral neuropathy and also lumbosacral radiculopathy. For now, let us only know that these are all classified as neurological disorders. This means that these disorders are a result of some malfunction in the nervous system. The way the messages are transmitted or translated is interrupted, causing an uncontrollable urge to move the limb.

The reflexes of the spinal cord, the spine flexor in particular, are controlled by certain mechanisms generated by a neurotransmitter called dopamine. So, dopamine is one of the key elements in the study of the pathophysiology of this condition and also its cure. If you have visited a doctor or have done any research about Restless Leg Syndrome, you would have heard the term "dopamine agonist" being used quite often. A dopamine agonist is a drug which stimulates certain parts of the brain and the nervous system. These activated areas are called receptors. These receptors are otherwise stimulated by the neurotransmitter dopamine. This is why dopamine medication is considered to be the most effective one in dealing with Restless Leg Syndrome. However, when the reports of the studies conducted were scrutinised, the results observed were quite mixed. In some cases, the synaptic activity or the transmission of neurological signals were considerably reduced. In other cases, there was no difference from the control group.

There have also been some studies which use dopamine antagonists. These drugs have an effect exactly opposite to dopamine agonists. These drugs block the receptor sites. When these drugs are administered, the symptoms of Restless Leg Syndrome go through the roof!

In addition to this, the proteins that are involved in the production of dopamine have a circadian rhythm. This means that these proteins are processed and utilised in a cycle that lasts 24 hours. If you look at the symptoms of RLS, even these symptoms are repeated in a certain cycle. You will experience the symptoms every 24 hours, usually. So, most researchers believe that a drop in the level of dopamine is the primary cause for Restless Leg Syndrome. These studies bring us to yet another cross road in the research about RLS. A similar mechanism is also observed in another disease called Parkinson's disease. The treatment methods are also very similar. So, it is believed that there could be some distinct association between the two conditions. While the causal factor is believed to be similar, this relationship could also be a breakthrough in finding a cure for the condition.

We will go into the details of the association between proteins, iron and RLS symptoms. However, for now, let us look at the basics as we cannot complete the pathophysiology without understanding this. The synthesis of iron and proteins is cyclic. It follows the 24 hour rhythm which makes it possible to associate them with RLS. Iron is a responsible for the production of an enzyme called tyrosine hydroxylase. This enzyme is responsible for limiting the rate at which dopamine is produced in our body. Naturally, when there is a dip in the level of iron, there is also a drop in the production of dopamine.

There have been many studies conducted on animals that have iron deficiency. In these animals, it was observed that the receptors of dopamine reduced in number. There was also an evident decrease in dopamine function. The density of dopamine transporters also decreased. However there was an elevation in the dopamine itself. This is a contradictory observation. But, what we know for sure is that the body's inability to access dopamine is the cause for RLS. The association between iron and this dopamine dysfunction is still to be studied in detail and proved.

Chapter 3: Diagnosing Restless Leg Syndrome

One of the biggest problems with Restless Leg Syndrome is its diagnosis. There is very little information available to understand this condition. Even with experienced doctors, most of the symptoms of RLS can go unrecognised. The reason is not lack of facility; it is basically a lack of research and knowledge about the condition itself. Since it is becoming more common in the current scenario, there has been a considerable amount of research that helps doctors diagnose the condition and provide necessary treatment.

1. Onset of the Condition

There are two types of Restless Leg Syndrome depending upon the age of onset of the condition. With RLS, there is no distinct age when the condition appears. It can affect toddlers, adolescents and adults. The question is: Why does the age of the patient matter?

Well, to begin with, the diagnosis of the treatment is different with children and with adults. Like I mentioned in the previous chapter, diagnosis in children is harder as you cannot understand the symptoms entirely. In addition to this, the mode of treatment may also vary as per the age of the person affected. The causal factors may vary between toddlers and adults and therefore, the mode of treatment is also drastically different. Usually, the diagnosis and treatment is the same for adolescents and adults. That means, if the person suffering from the condition is 13 years or older, the method of treatment is most probably the same.

There two kinds of RLS based on the onset are:

Early Onset: As the name suggests, Early Onset means that the symptoms of the condition become apparent when the person is

12 years old or younger. For most individuals, onset of RLS is early. Of course, it is the diagnosis which may go wrong leading to complications later on in life. With early onset, it has been observed that one parent or some member in the family usually has this condition. So, this means that the condition is genetic. Therefore, the treatment can be more elaborate. While home remedies can provide temporary relief, you need to provide elaborate treatment to ensure that the condition does not get worse as the age progresses. Other factors leading to early onset are the diet and nutrition of the child.

Late Onset: Late Onset means that the symptoms begin to appear when the individual is over 13 years of age. The symptoms most likely occur in the legs and the lower back when the onset is late. It is not necessary for the individual to have a family history of Restless Leg Syndrome. Usually the condition is neurological when the onset of the condition is later. This means that the nervous system could be damaged or might have degenerated due to age. It could also be because of nutrient deficiency and a poor lifestyle.

Research to understand the distinct characteristics of Late and Early Onset

A recently published medical report provided the details of a research conducted to understand early and late onset of Restless Leg Syndrome in greater detail. The objective of this research was to understand the distribution of the age of onset among a large population. In the process, the clinical characteristics of individuals with early and late onset were compared. This provided more data to enable better treatment and diagnosis of the condition based on the onset.

The study was conducted on 250 individuals with RLS. The data that was collected dealt with various important aspects of the condition. All the necessary information about age of onset, the history of diseases in the family, the severity of the condition and also the symptoms was collected. Special interest was paid to the age of onset as that was the objective of this study. They estimated the density of various factors using special statistical methods. The outcome of the study was rather interesting.

The results of the age of onset were bimodal. In statistics, there are two types of distribution of data. The first one is unimodal which means that the density of the data is highest at a certain value. The second one is called bimodal. In this type of distribution, the density is maximum at two points. So when represented graphically, you will notice two distinct peaks in the results of the study.

Even with Restless Leg Syndrome, there were two such distinct peaks with respect to the age of onset. The first peak was observed at the age of 20 while the second one was observed in the mid-40s. With these statistics, there was a separating cut off of 36 years between early onset and late onset of the condition.

There were also several differences in the distribution of the age of onset with respect to the etiology and the family history of the condition. If you remember, we discussed primary and secondary RLS in the previous chapters. The distinction between these two types of RLS is also seen with the age of onset. Primary RLS usually has an early onset of the symptoms while secondary RLS usually has a late onset of the symptoms.

There were other notable differences between the two conditions. With early onset of RLS the periodic leg movements during sleep is higher. There are also instances of small symptoms or microarousals along with limb movements during wakefulness with early onset. The entire pathological process of the two conditions is significantly different between the two groups. With the early onset group the condition is determined genetically while there are several other ways of determining it with late onset. It is also possible to distinguish between the two conditions based on the history of the disease in the family.

Since these two conditions are so distinct, the diagnosis is also significantly different. The commonality between them is the determining factors that make the diagnosis of Restless Leg Syndrome definite, possible or probable.

2. Definite, Possible and Probable

Definite Diagnosis

With definite diagnosis, there are two possibilities. The criteria in both the possibilities are same for adults and children. There are four criteria that the adult or child must confirmed in order to provide a definite diagnosis of the condition.

Possibility 1

The following four criteria should be confirmed:

- There is a strong urge to move the legs as there is relief from the symptoms
- When the individual is lying down or resting, the need to move the legs.
- This urge to move diminishes completely or partially when the person begins to move around.
- Usually, the movement of the limbs becomes worse at night or towards the evening. It may occur during the day and get worse towards the evening. It is also possible that the symptoms occur exclusively towards evening or at night.

In addition to the above criteria, the individual also complains of a lot of discomfort in the legs. This is in the form of cramps or even extreme pain. In case of children, they may use their own words to describe the sensations as creepies, tickles, bugs and even too much energy in the limbs.

Possibility 2

The second possibility for a definite diagnosis of Restless Leg Syndrome is also available. This second possibility is usually applied with children. The first step to this diagnosis is

determining and confirming the four criteria mentioned above. In addition to that, the child must also comply with two or all three of the following supportive criteria:
- The sleep disturbance for the age of the child can be clinically determined.
- One of the biological parents or the sibling of the child has definite Restless Leg Syndrome.
- When a sleep study is conducted, the periodic limb movement index is at least 5 or more for every hour of sleep.

With definite diagnosis, the next step is treatment of the condition. There is no need to look for other symptoms or conduct other tests when the criteria required have been met with.

Probable Diagnosis

Even with probable diagnosis, there are two possibilities. When you have a probable diagnosis, you may have to conduct a few more tests or check the response of the individual to the treatment provided to confirm the condition. With this type of diagnosis, it is not possible to be 100% sure that the condition is RLS and nothing else. However, there is enough reason to suspect that the individual is suffering from Restless Leg Syndrome.

Possibility 1

The individual must meet the three conditions mentioned below:
- There is a strong urge to move the limbs, usually the legs.
- The need to move the leg either starts or becomes worse when the individual is resting or simply lying down.
- This strong urge to move is relieved totally or partially when the person actually moves.

In addition to this, there is a biological parent, sibling or some family member who has been diagnosed with definite RLS. If you have noticed, in case of a probable diagnosis of the condition, the cycle of the symptoms does not occur. They may manifest themselves at any time of the day and at any intervals. Sometimes, the symptoms may be absent for several days before recurring. The intensity may also vary quite significantly.

Possibility 2

Again the second possibility is mostly with children. You must be observant of when the symptoms aggravate. Usually, there is great discomfort in the lower part of the body when the child is lying down or sitting. There may be violent motor movements of the area that has been affected. These movements could be voluntary or involuntary. The child also shows the characteristic criteria mentioned above. These symptoms become worse in a state of complete inactivity. Also, the symptoms are immediately relieved with movement. Sometimes, these symptoms may exhibit a certain pattern of occurrence. Just like any adult symptom, even these symptoms occurring in the child could be maximum towards the evening or at nightfall. If the child has a biological parent or a family member who has been diagnosed with definite Restless Leg Syndrome, you could make a probable diagnosis. In this case, if you notice the symptoms mentioned above may or may not occur. When they do, they tend to be cyclic and quite distinct.

Possible Diagnosis

There are only two criteria to make a possible diagnosis of Restless Leg Syndrome. A possible diagnosis usually occurs in children and infants when it is difficult to determine the sensations and the symptoms experienced by the child. Possible diagnosis is the first step to understanding if the child may have sleep issues or even behavioural issues due to Restless Leg Syndrome. When you notice that the child is not able to focus or is showing disruptive behaviour due to lack of sleep, a possible diagnosis can help you provide the right treatment.

For a possible diagnosis, the child must show periodic leg movements. This may occur when the child is resting or even when the child has fallen asleep. These movements tend to occur at intervals of 30seconds to 1 minute. In any case, if you can see periodic movements of the limbs 5 times or more every hour of sleep, it is possible that the child has RLS. In addition to this, if the child has a parent or a sibling who has definite RLS, then you might want to consider this condition as the primary cause of sleeplessness.

Whether it is a definite, possible or probable diagnosis, you must never ignore the chances of an individual having Restless Leg Syndrome. It is only when the signs are ignored that the condition can become terrible enough to interfere with the life of the individual. You must also understand that the effects of Restless Leg Syndrome are not restricted to the physical space. One is also affected emotionally and psychologically to a very large extent. If you read the testimonies of people suffering from this condition, you will realise that the latter are actually of greater concern than the condition itself.

Other Diagnosis possibilities

These days doctors often do a Doppler Study Test. This is to rule out Peripheral Arterial Disease - a condition affecting the arteries and blood flow through your body. The test involves laying on a bed for approx. 20 minutes whilst your blood pressure in your ankles/feet is compared to the blood pressure in your upper arms. It is a non invasive test and the person doing the test uses a small hand held device and holds it against your skin, on different places, reading the results from a little monitor.

If the Doppler Study Test is normal, a Nerve Conduction Test can also be carried out. This test measures how quickly electrical signals move in your body, through a particular peripheral nerve. It is a non invasive test : electrodes are placed on your skin and the person doing the test will view the results on a computer screen. The test can feel slightly uncomfortable but is not painful. This test will find any damage to the peripheral nervous system.

3. Diagnosis in Children and Toddlers

When the onset of Restless Leg Syndrome is early, then you have three steps to diagnose the condition. Each step is important as it can help make a definite, possible or probable diagnosis. Here are the three diagnostic measures taken with children:

Take a thorough family history

We will go into the genetics of RLS in the following sections. At this point, it is important to understand that RLS presents a dominant inheritance pattern. This means if one of the biological parent is suffering from RLS, then there is a 50:50 chance that the condition will be passed on to one or all of his or her children. In many cases, even the initial diagnosis of the parent's condition happens only when the child's symptoms are being studied. Therefore, the first step of diagnosis of this condition is having an elaborate interview of the parents about possible RLS symptoms that they may be experiencing. If they meet the criteria listed in the previous section, then, there is a possibility that the condition has been inherited.

Conduct a physical examination

In a child who shows the symptoms of Restless Leg Syndrome, it is normal to have a thorough physical examination. Usually, in case of children, there are fewer chances of underlying medical issues that are causing the symptoms of RLS. The only thing that is noticed in case of childhood RLS is iron deficiency. Other problems like neuropathy, failure of the kidneys and diabetes is less common in children. However, there are chances that these conditions also occur. Hence, physical examination becomes an important step in determining the treatment that can solve the issue and control the symptoms to a large extent.

Conducting a sleep test

The most obvious symptoms of Restless Leg Syndrome are observed when a child is asleep. Most often, Restless Leg Syndrome and Periodic Limb Movements are categorised as "restlessness" and inability to sleep in case of children. So, a sleep study is necessary to check for the actual causes of the sleeping issues in the child.

The scientific name of a sleep study is a polysomnography. If your doctor recommends this, do not be alarmed. It is just an attempt to check the sleep pattern of the child. The procedure is very simple. However, it is not enough to just observe the child when he or she is asleep. There are certain "readings" that need to be taken in order to provide a diagnosis that is accurate. So, you will have to take your child to a proper sleep center.

When you are choosing a sleep centre for your child make sure you opt for one that has ample experience in dealing with children. They must use the proper techniques to study the sleep patterns of the child. The score that is obtained at the end of a test is very important in determining whether the child has RLS or not.

4. Diagnosis in Adults

For those of you who are still understanding the condition that is Restless Leg Syndrome, it might be surprising to know that there is a separate Medical Advisory Board for Restless Leg Syndrome. The main purpose of this board is to provide all the criteria that are necessary in classifying the symptoms of Restless Leg Syndrome. In case of adults, treatment decisions are made based on whether Restless Leg Syndrome is intermittent or daily. In case of intermittent RLS, the condition is serious and troublesome enough to get medical attention. However, daily therapy is not necessary as the symptoms do not occur every day. On the other hand, in case of daily RLS, the symptoms are so severe that the individual needs to be treated on a daily basis.

The first step towards the quantification of the condition in adults is checking the sleep pattern in a proper sleep laboratory. If the limb movements and the symptoms occur five times and over in an hour of sleep, then it is considered an anomaly. That is when diagnosing Restless Leg Syndrome is warranted.

Here, it is important to note that periodic limb movements are not the only criteria for RLS. There are other tests that need to be conducted in order to confirm the condition. Some common tests are polysomnography and actigraphy. These tests help determine if the person has Restless Leg Syndrome or whether he is suffering only from periodic leg movements.

In case of adults, there are several other conditions that can be confused with Restless Leg Syndrome. Even simple leg cramps are wrongly diagnosed sometimes. There are more serious conditions like nocturnal recumbence and akathisia that need a different type of treatment altogether. These conditions cause more painful contractions in the muscle. The pain is very focused in these conditions. The first instances of confusion between akathisia and Restless Leg Syndrome were observed in the mid-20th century when neuroleptic drugs were introduced. These medications caused restlessness in the limbs followed by a need to move the limbs in patients who consumed them. However, this condition is quite different from Restless Leg Syndrome in its pathology and symptoms.

In some cases, the symptoms of Restless Leg Syndrome in adults are caused by medication. This is when a physical examination becomes crucial. Certain medicines that contain serotonin inhibitors, caffeine or lithium may cause symptoms similar to Restless Leg Syndrome.

For instance, when serotonin inhibitors are consumed, they tend to increase the serotonin levels in the body. This also results in changes in the dopamine levels in the body. Several studies have been conducted on animals to determine the effects of lithium. According to these studies, the dopamine release and also the number of receptors of dopamine are altered when the lithium levels in the body are not balanced. When lithium intake is high, dopamine levels are compromised. Therefore, RLS symptoms are observed.

The last thing you need to understand in case of adults is whether there are any peripheral neuropathies. These neuropathies may also occur when the individual has diabetes or other conditions. The symptoms that are displayed are very similar to RLS. This is when the four criteria to confirm RLS become important.

You see diseases like diabetes and other vascular diseases produce symptoms that are very similar to RLS. So, in case of adults, a thorough peripheral vascular exam, study of peripheral pules and physical examination to determine the presence of any ulcers is necessary. Doctors may even conduct examination of physical traits like distribution of hair on the legs to confirm if it is some other condition altogether which is leading to Restless Leg Syndrome. Doctors often will also do a Nerve Conduction Test.

My diagnosis:

- First my doctor did a Doppler Study Test. In my case, the result of the test was that my flood flow was normal and I did not suffer from Peripheral Arterial Disease.

- Next, my doctor tested my reflexes (with a small hammer) and concluded that my reflexes in my legs were *not* normal. He referred me to a neurologist to have a Nerve Conduction Study. The result of that was that my nerves were *not* responding normally, causing my RLS. Medication is the only option, the neurologist said. I have not started my medication yet and will postpone it as long as I can.

Medication I have been prescribed:

- Gabapentin 300mg Capsules - take 2 at night.

- Pramipexole Dihydrochloride - 125mg - take 1 at night.

Chapter 4: Living with Restless Leg Syndrome

Once the condition has been diagnosed, the next thing you need to prepare yourself for is actually living with the condition. There are several parallel effects of the condition that can alter the quality of your life. The effects extend to various spheres of your life. There are several treatments and home remedies that are available for you to seek relief from the condition. But, what is more important is that you know exactly what to expect along the course of treatment.

I find this chapter to be of maximum importance as people tend to respond poorly to the treatment as the condition can take complete control of your routine. Knowing what is in store helps you find methods to deal with this condition.

First, you need to know that this is a very serious condition. I am not trying to scare you. However, the repercussions are a lot more intense than pain or cramps in the legs. The RLS foundation has changed the name of the condition to Willis Ekbom Disease to provide a proper method to diagnose and treat the condition.

If you have been diagnosed with the condition or whether you suspect that you have Restless Leg Syndrome, here are some pointers that can be of great help to you.

Never self-diagnose the condition

It is true that there are four distinct criteria that will help you determine whether the condition is, in fact, RLS or not. So, if you think that you just have to observe your symptoms and you will know what you have, you are wrong. Sometimes the symptoms itself are very vague and confusing. Even if you are entirely certain that you are suffering from RLS, make sure you go to a sleep center or visit a doctor for a more accurate diagnosis of the condition.

Sleeplessness

The sensations that you experience in your legs, arms or back, can be similar or can vary from day to day. Many of my personal contacts who suffer from Restless Leg Syndrome describe the feeling similarly. They say that it feels like someone is poking them with a stick at short intervals when they are trying to fall asleep. I can relate to this too. The worst thing is that it does not matter how tired or exhausted you are. Your body will wake you up and make you walk around or move around even if you are not mentally up to it. Just imagine this. You have come home after an all-nighter. All you want to do is fall asleep and you have construction workers turning on a jackhammer. All this, every single day! Can you relate to the frustrating feeling?

Always feeling fidgety

If you have RLS along with periodic limb movement, it is not enough to just take regular sleep medication. Even if you have been entirely knocked out by a certain medicine, your limbs will continue to move without your voluntary involvement. This may not happen only when one is trying to fall asleep. It may happen when you are in the passenger seat of a car, taking a long ride on the subway or even when you are out watching movies. This is when it becomes mandatory to take your medicines along with you wherever you go. If not, people who are not aware of your condition might be excessively annoyed. Besides that, it is also extremely embarrassing to have your legs flying about without any control.

Allergies can be excruciating

In case you suffer from seasonal allergies, you have all the more reasons to be worried about your condition. Sometimes, you could also be allergic to a pet in your home when it begins to shed fur. The common thing to do is to take an antihistamine medicine that will prevent allergic reactions. However, these medications can aggravate the symptoms of Restless Leg Syndrome to a large extent. None the less, not taking the medication means that you will have a severe allergic reaction that can be damaging.

This is when you need to weigh the severity of the RLS symptoms with the allergies. Many times, individuals are not aware of this. So, they may be able to detect a pattern in their RLS symptoms which tend to spike in the allergy season. But, they may not know that it is their allergy medicines that are causing the severe symptoms.

You will think twice before massages

I know I do and so do several other individuals suffering from RLS. A hot stone massage, especially, is nothing close to the luxury that it is for most people. When a hot stone is placed on the pressure points, the uncontrollable need to move may arise. This is when you have to literally clinch all the muscles to make sure that the stones do not go flying across the room. Even if the person at the spa tells you that it is the toxins that are causing the reaction, for a person suffering from RLS, the cause is well known. It is okay for you to go out and get a massage. You may not have any reaction at all. However, this is to help you understand what may happen when you go out for a relaxing massage. Remember, relaxing aggravates the symptoms.

Alcohol alert

Any substance that can cause an alteration in your sleep pattern must be kept at a good distance. We know that caffeine is usually the culprit. However, alcohol, which is expected to induce sleep, can have reverse effects when you have Restless Leg Syndrome. Personally, I feel that even a glass of red wine can make my symptoms go haywire and just keep me up all night. While all these effects of RLS could seem terrible, the good news is that treatment is available. You must always visit a doctor when you notice initial symptoms or even a variation in the symptoms after you have been diagnosed with the condition.

Chapter 5: Who is Most Prone?

The funny thing about Restless Leg Syndrome is that it is a very common condition. I find this funny because considering the frequency it can be labelled as one of the most underdiagnosed conditions that affect our society.

According to various studies that have been conducted globally, it has been noted that Restless Leg Syndrome is not so common in the Asian Population. In the rest of the world, at least 10% of the entire population is affected by Restless Leg Syndrome.

The studies conducted are across age groups and also between the two genders. In a recent study, telephonic interviews were conducted on a random population. The study was localised in Kentucky and the size of the group was 1803. It was noted that the prevalence of the condition was in 10% of the population.

Another similar study was conducted in Canada. In this study, the objective was to understand which gender is more affected by this condition. The observation was that RLS symptoms were seen in 17% of the women and in 13% of the men. The size of this group was 2019 individuals. Globally, the statistics reveal that women are more prone to this condition than men. In fact it is twice as prevalent in women as it is in men. There are several reasons for this including the fact that RLS is observed during pregnancy and also because women tend to be affected more by emotional trauma.

In Europe, extensive studies have been conducted in Germany. In one such survey on a group of 4000 people, the overall prevalence was noted to be 10.6%. In this survey, the interviews were conducted face to face and a standard set of questions were used to score the individuals. In places like Rothdach, the prevalence was about 9.8%. This study was conducted on a group of 370 participants who were in the age group of 65 to 83 years.

Coming to the Asian countries, there are a few studies that have been conducted in Japan. The most important one was conducted on urban residents of Japan. The group consisted of about 4600 participants. In this study only one symptom of RLS was targeted. The questionnaire was self-administered. There were just two questions. One was about the sleep disturbance and the other was about the need to move the legs around because of the sensations. The scored revealed that between the age group of 20 and 29, 3% of the women were affected. With an age group of 50 to 59 years of age, the prevalence was about 7%.

The scores were quite contrary to the ones obtained in non-Asian countries. These scores revealed that Restless Leg Syndrome was more common in men than in the women. A major difference related to gender in the prevalence was noticed in the age group of men between 49 to 49 years of age. In men, however, the symptoms had no relationship with the age of the individual.

In a premium healthcare centre in Singapore the data collected showed that the prevalence was much lesser. The study was conducted on individuals aged 21 years and above. The size of the group was 1000 individuals. The population was predominantly Asian. It was noted that only 0.6% of the male population showed the symptoms of Restless Leg Syndrome. In the women, the prevalence was just 0.1%.

What was observed in all these studies is that in the Asian and American studies, the gender difference was not so obvious. However, in the German studies, women were more affected by the condition than men. The Canadian study also showed that restlessness at night was higher in women than in the men.

These studies look at the prevalence of the condition among populations. However, there are several factors that determine who is more prone to the condition. People who are anaemic are susceptible to Restless Leg Syndrome. Other nutritional factors are also important. This includes magnesium and lithium consumption as well.

Women may develop symptoms of restless leg syndrome when they are pregnant. The hormonal changes that take place may give way to RLS.

The familial history also has an important role to play. Since RLS is genetic in nature, early onset is usually linked to the occurrence of the condition in the family. Even with late onset, the possibilities are higher if there is a family history of Restless Leg Syndrome.

The occurrence of Restless Leg Syndrome is also more probable when you consume certain medication. These medicines may have an effect on the production of neurotransmitters that are responsible for your sleep patterns. If you are on hormone therapy, as well, you are susceptible to this condition.

Neurological damage with age can lead to symptoms of Restless Leg Syndrome. It can also occur due to conditions like diabetes.

Besides all these factors, you must also consider environmental factors like substance abuse, work stress etc. as they can affect sleep patterns. In case of substance abuse, when you are trying to get off the substance, Restless Leg Syndrome can occur as a withdrawal symptom.

So you see, when you look at the statistics available, it seems like there should be a lot more information on the condition itself. However, including the causal factors, very little is known about Restless Leg Syndrome.

Chapter 6: Diseases That Are Mistaken For RLS

The symptoms of Restless Leg Syndrome are very similar to other neurological conditions. Sometimes, the smallest pinching sensation in the legs is considered RLS. I have been at the receiving end of statements like: "Sitting for long hours gives me cramps, I must have restless leg syndrome." of "My legs feel horrible when I lay down". These careless statements can be difficult for a person who is actually working through the condition.

However, there are also serious conditions like Parkinson's disease that have similar causal factors and very similar pathology. The treatment is drastically different which makes it important to know how to differentiate between these conditions.

1. PLMD v/s RLS

Periodic Limb Movement Disorder and Restless Leg Syndrome are extremely similar. However, these are two distinct disorders. The reason it is difficult to differentiate between these diseases is because they often occur together. If you have Restless Leg Syndrome, you will have a good chance of having Periodic Limb Movements. However, the reverse is false.

Like you know already, with RLS, there are several uncomfortable sensations in the legs. These sensations tend to occur mostly at night. You will feel like kicking your legs about in order to get some relief from the symptoms. In case of PLMD, a person kicks his legs around and also jerks his arms involuntarily all night long. These movements might occur hundreds of times on some nights. Most often, the individual is not even aware of the fact that his limbs have been moving all night.

40

There are many key differences between the two conditions. For most people who have Restless Leg Syndrome, iron deficiency is quite common. If you can take iron supplements on a regular basis, not only is iron deficiency treated, but the symptoms of RLS also reduce considerably. This is not true for individuals who are suffering from PLMD.

Sleep deprivation is more severe in case of Restless Leg Syndrome. This is because the symptoms occur in when you are awake and prevent you from falling asleep. On the other hand, with PLMD, it is possible to be woken up for a few minutes because of the sudden symptoms. However, it is possible to fall asleep.

The movements in case of RLS are voluntary. You need to move to ease the symptoms. With PLMD, you may not even be aware of the symptoms. Sometimes, the episodes of movement may prolong for several hours. The nature of the condition makes diagnosis itself different. Since you are aware of the symptoms in case of RLS, it is possible for you to start the diagnosis with a simple description of the symptoms. In case of PLMD, it is necessary to study the sleep pattern of the person. This requires you to enrol yourself at a professional sleep clinic. Most often, the individual will seek assistance only when a partner or maybe a parent complains of these sudden and rather violent movements. Therefore, it is possible for PLMD to go unnoticed for several years on end.

2. RLS v/s Parkinson's disease

The commonality between RLS and Parkinson's disease is that they are both neurological conditions. They both respond to therapy that is dopaminergic. The relationship between the two conditions has not been entirely explored, however. But, there is a good chance that individuals with Parkinson's disease may display symptoms of Restless Leg Syndrome. The surveys that have been conducted often include individuals with Parkinson's disease who have observed symptoms of RLS. There have also been several comparisons between individuals who have PD with individuals who have only RLS.

These studies have revealed that there is a higher chance of occurrence of RLS in individuals who have Parkinson's disease. So far, there is very little understanding of the risk involved when patients with Parkinson's disease also develop Restless Leg Syndrome. It is possible to say that RLS is actually one of the symptoms of Parkinson's disease. In case of Parkinson's there are several other sensory and motor symptoms that could easily be confused with RLS. Also, the symptoms of RLS are a lot milder when they are observed in a patient with Parkinson's disease.

The response to therapy is also significantly different between individuals with RLS and Parkinson's. In the former condition, when any dopaminergic therapy is provided, the symptoms may increase drastically in the initial stages. The symptoms also vary in their occurrence. They may begin to appear earlier and can also be distributed to other parts of the body. In case of patients with Parkinson's disease, new symptoms may develop. This includes motor fluctuations as well. The complications of treatment are fewer in case of patients with RLS.

Another major difference lies in the iron content. In case of RLS, the symptoms are a result of iron deficiency. So, taking iron tablets can reduce the symptoms considerably. On the other hand, in case of individuals with PD, the iron levels have been observed to be quite contrary. The levels of iron and ferritin in certain regions of the nervous system increase. This causes oxidative stress which is the primary cause of degeneration of dopamine in the body leading to symptoms of Parkinson's.

MRI scans have revealed that the level of iron in the same region of the nervous system was significantly lesser in case of patients with Restless Leg Syndrome. These differences were also confirmed by several neuropathological studies.

When you look at the similarities in the two conditions, it is possible to say that there must be some relationship between them. Although they are different in their pathology and also the diagnostic criteria, it is the dopamine levels that form the underlying factor to link these two conditions. Although the mechanism of the anomaly is different with both the conditions, it is this neurotransmitter that plays a very important role. Of course, there is no evidence to confirm that there is any role of genetics in linking these two conditions. The pathological mechanisms of the conditions themselves are not entirely known to provide any concrete link between RLS and PLMD.

3. RLS v/s Akathisia

Many doctors may mislead you saying that akathisia and RLS are two different names for the same condition. Even online, you will be able to find several sources that will vouch that akathisia is the medical name for RLS. You must always remember that the medical name for this condition is Willis Ekbom Disease. Akathisia is an entirely different condition that was mistaken for RLS after a drug that was released in the mid-20th century. This medicine produced RLS like symptoms as a side effect, making many believe that they two conditions are the same.

The name Akathisia is derived from a Greek word which means "not sitting still". This condition is characterised by extreme restlessness, making it similar to RLS. But the two conditions are extremely different right from their pathology to the symptoms experienced by the individual. In case of akathisia, there may be an uncontrollable need to move the limbs. The movements are rather obvious and violent and are usually restricted to the lower limb. This is the first diagnostic criteria for RLS. Therefore, it is natural to have these two conditions mixed up.

The symptoms exhibited in case of akathisia are far more intense. They also have several underlying psychological factors that lead to the need to move the limbs violently. The symptoms can be so severe in case of this disease that it may drive an individual to the point of committing suicide. Besides these, serious urges towards violence and even homicide occur when an individual suffers from akathisia. This condition is most often medication induced. When a person consumes high doses of tranquilisers or even drugs, akathasia may manifest itself as a side effect of this condition. Although there are several instances of medical induced RLS, it is important to know that these two conditions are poles apart.

To begin with, the symptoms of akathisia may be similar to RLS. However, the bigger differentiator is the fact that akathisia does not follow a circadian cycle. So, it may occur at any time of the day. In case of RLS, the symptoms aggravate towards night or evening. It may also become severe when the person is resting. Moving actually eases the symptoms in case of RLS. However, this is not true for akathisia. While the symptoms may reduce with movement, they are persistent, constant and very difficult to treat.

The movements in case of akathisia can also be involuntary sometimes. For instance, a person who is standing can suddenly start marching on the spot. This movement is not an attempt to eliminate the symptoms. It is completely involuntary. It is not necessary for a person to be at rest for the symptoms of akathisia to occur. Because of these differences in the stimuli and triggers, the treatment of the two conditions differs a lot. One major distinction is that dopaminergic is usually not recommended for akathisia. In case of RLS, this treatment is viewed as the core for treating the condition.

4. RLS v/s Nocturnal Cramps

Sometimes, we may experience nocturnal leg cramps when we are asleep. Although these cramps are, very often, confused with RLS, the two conditions are entirely different.

In case of nocturnal leg cramps, the muscles in the leg, mostly the calf region, are primarily affected. These muscles cramp causing pain and discomfort. On the other hand, in case or RLS, the symptoms may extend to other body parts as well. But, as for nocturnal cramps, the will never manifest in any other part of the body besides the legs.

When cramps occur, the sensations can be very painful. There is no tingling or creeping feeling, however. You can be relieved from these sensations by walking around or stretching. But, the most effective way to get rid of nocturnal cramps is to press down on the foot really hard. While moving around works really well in case of RLS symptoms, pressing the leg down hard can cause an increase in the intensity of the symptoms.

When you experience leg cramps, the muscles are actually contracted. The pain will last for more than 20 seconds. There is no specific type of leg movement, however. The muscle activation in case of Restless Leg Syndrome is for smaller durations. These spurts occur for less than 10 seconds but can repeat themselves frequently. Leg cramps will only occur when you are lying down. However, RLS symptoms may be executed even when the person is sitting down or relaxing.

While leg cramps tend to last for longer intervals, you can expect the symptoms to go away and not recur for the rest of the night. RLS will repeat itself rather rapidly, causing extreme sleep deprivation and discomfort for late hours into the night.

The symptoms of RLS, like you know well by now, will occur with an interval of 24 hours, usually at night. With leg cramps, there is no cycle, per say. These symptoms are most likely to occur after you have fallen asleep, usually when you are in the REM state of sleep. The most common occurrence of cramps is early in the morning. This is when the symptoms of RLS begin to diminish. The treatment for the two conditions is significantly different. In case of RLS, the symptoms can be reduced with effective iron deficiency treatment. This is, however, of no use in case of individuals with nocturnal leg cramps. In fact, there are no common medicines that have been used to treat RLS and nocturnal leg cramps.

In fact, leg cramps can be resolved easily and spontaneously with some stretches. In some severe cases,   quinine is used as an effective treatment option. Several studies using control groups have determined that quinine can significantly reduce the occurrence of nocturnal cramps. However, the use of quinine also has serious side effects. In some patients it can also cause loss of vision and, in worst cases, fatality due to toxic reactions. So when you compare the benefits with the risks, this is still a questionable method of treating nocturnal cramps. In case of RLS, quinine is not an option at all.

The only possible similarity between these two conditions is that they have the potential to cause serious sleep deprivation. You may also count the fact that the two conditions affect the limbs. Besides these two factors, there are absolutely no similarities between these conditions. They are pathologically different. The symptoms and their occurrence also vary. Therefore, correct diagnosis is necessary to provide the right treatment for the condition that actually exists.

5. RLS v/s ADHD

It is very common to confuse RLS with Attention Deficit Hyperactivity Disorder. In case of symptoms that occur during the day, RLS is usually wrongly diagnosed as ADHD as there is difficulty in sitting in one place for a long period of time. This wrong diagnosis usually occurs in case of children in a classroom set up. They are considered to have ADHD as they tend to move around and even disturb the class. In many cases, RLS is believed to be a psychological disorder that is causing bad behaviour in the child. The truth is that RLS is actually a neurological condition that requires great care and attention.

Children have been sent to special schools and have also been started off on treatment for ADHD because of misdiagnosis. Yes, there is a possibility that the two conditions are related. It is possible for a child who has ADHD to have symptoms of RLS. In fact, some studies have revealed that 44% of individuals with

ADHD show RLS symptoms. However, it is not necessary that a child with RLS needs psychological care. Less than 20% of children with RLS have ADHD. There is very little information available to understand the link between the two conditions. All the evaluations that have been conducted so far reveal that sleep deprivation is one of the primary causes for this type of misdiagnosis. When a child is unable to sleep because of RLS, he tends to be irritable and even aggressive when he is awake. Children also tend to have impaired cognitive function because of sleep deprivation. This make them slow learners in addition to being inattentive. This is pointed out as bad behaviour.

The only way to differentiate between the two conditions is a reference to the diagnostic criteria for Restless Leg Syndrome. Most often, a child with ADHD will not comply with even one criterion, thus ruling out ADHD. Another reason for this confusion is the fact that the two conditions respond to dopaminergic treatments. But, these two conditions are entirely different. The primary difference is the fact that one is psychological while the other is neuropathic.

Now you can see why there is so much confusion in the medical world about the treatment of RLS. Therefore, several home remedies have cropped up to provide temporary relief from the symptoms. Of course, before treatment, you must know what causes the condition. When you get to the root of this, better diagnosis and treatment will become possible.

Chapter 7: What Causes RLS?

For the last 20 years, there has been extensive research with respect to RLS. These studies have shown that RLS may have several causal factors depending on whether it is primary or secondary. Although the research is extensive, the problem with RLS is that most often the exact causal factors are idiopathic. This means that the exact factors are seldom known.

According to one doctor, RLS is simply the sign of degeneration or dying off of our legs. Our ancestors used their legs extensively. They even ran on four legs for centuries. We hardly ever run on our two legs now! We sit all day and when we walk, we usually walk on our heels, which is wrong. So the use of the legs has changed drastically in the modern times. For this reason, our heart and brain lasts longer than our legs and feet. Most people say that their left leg is worse than their right leg. This is because, when we drive the car, our right foot gets more exercise.

This is one hypothesis but there are several possible causes for RLS that is still not fully known. This is why the diagnosis of this condition is extensive and quite elaborate. In this chapter we will discuss all the probable causes of RLS.

1.The Role of Dopamine

Dopamine is a neurotransmitter which is produced in the neurons present in the brain. A neurotransmitter is a type of messenger that takes the information or the signals from one neuron to the other. Now, dopamine is one of the most controversial neurotransmitters which have divided the entire scientific communities into several groups that are trying to understand the exact function of this chemical in our brain.

All that they know of this neurotransmitter definitely is that it has the ability to control most of our behaviour patterns. It is very important for several regulatory functions. However, despite its importance in the body, it is not produced in large volumes. Only 0.3% of all the neurons present in the brain produce this neurotransmitter. Some of these neurons are present in a section of our nervous system called substantia nigra.

Until I began my research on dopamine and its effects on RLS, I was very ignorant of the power that this chemical has on us. Until very recently, I used to blame the will power of drug addicts and substance abusers. In my opinion, the fact that they used the drugs continually, despite knowing the consequences was unacceptable. This was before I realised that dopamine can play a major role in controlling the urges.

You see, one of the most important functions of dopamine is reward recognition. Whenever we encounter a positive experience, dopamine is released. So, most often, it could just be this neurotransmitter which is responsible for the "nice" feeling that you have inside. So, this similar nice feeling is also experienced by drug users. Dopamine release causes pleasant sensations that we tend to remember. When a particular substance triggers the release of dopamine, we just want it more.

But, what does this have to do with RLS? It is definitely not a nice feeling! So, how does dopamine release connect with the rather unpleasant feelings and the hours of sleeplessness that we have to endure?

The answer lies in the fact that dopamine is also responsible for the regulation of sleep. For a long time, it was believed that only the enzymes melatonin and norepinephrine are responsible for our sleep cycle. But, research suggests that dopamine levels can determine the levels of melatonin as well. So when dopamine is produced in abundance, melatonin is blocked, making an individual awake and unable to fall asleep at all.

So, it must be that RLS is caused by excessive production of dopamine. Let us see what the studies say. The Cerebrospinal Fluid has been studied to understand the dopamine system in the body. While this is a rather crude method, the data proves the hypothesis that dopamine is actually high in individuals with RLS.

This means that dopamine therapy to reduce the levels of dopamine in the body should do the trick. But, drugs that block dopamine system actually cause reverse results. The symptoms are aggravated. With this contrast in the studies and the treatment, the need to explore deeper arose.

That is when the receptors of dopamine were studied. You see, the receptors are certain proteins that are able to lock or bind the dopamine. It is through this binding mechanism that dopamine is able to transmit the signals. Now, these proteins are fewer in numbers in individuals who have RLS.

Studies using the tissues of the brain showed that there was no physical damage to the receptor cells. It was the protein that was not available in the required amount. The study of the brain tissue also revealed that the protein responsible for triggering the production of dopamine was increased. This is what caused an increase in the level to this neurotransmitter.

Basically, the level of dopamine is high, but the response to lowering the level of dopamine is negative. This means that the body is functioning as if dopamine levels are low.

To help you understand this situation, let me give you a simple routine example. When you are watching TV and you are unable to hear the dialogues, what do you do? You just turn the volume up. Now the neurons had the signals but were unable to "hear" them are the receptors were low. So, they increase the production of dopamine to turn the "volume" up. Now, dopamine has an effect on the brain only at certain times of the day. This also explains the cyclic pattern of RLS.

What made the receptor concept clearer was the use of dopamine receptor agonists in treatment of RLS. These medicines activated the receptor sites and reduced the symptoms of Restless Syndrome. The next step that needs to be explored is the association between iron levels in our body and dopamine production. Since iron deficiency is the primary causal factor in RLS, it could be linked to protein production.

They only available studies involve the brain cell cultures of animals. These brain cells showed a significant change in the dopamine production when the iron levels were decreased. These studies have allowed us to create models. It is a possibility that these models could also be used to understand the actual function of dopamine and its relationship with iron in the human body. All we know for now is that dopamine therapy is one of the most important treatment options available. If we are able to link it to iron deficiency, we could find better ways of managing the condition.

2. The Role of Genetics

Our genetics can provide the answer to several diseases that we inherit. In some cases, the answers are rather simple as there is an obvious mutation in certain genes that cause a certain condition. For instance, in case of sickle celled anaemia, it is the damage to a specific gene that affects the body. Now our DNA is made of several proteins. With diseases with such obvious mutations, the proteins are either produced abnormally or are completely absent. So, these anomalies are much easier to detect. Sometimes, they can even be detected through tests and scans of a foetus.

The difficulty with understanding the role of genetics comes with conditions like Restless Leg Syndrome, Alzheimer's etc. With these conditions there is not just one obvious damaged gene. There is an interaction between several genes and also the environmental conditions. These diseases may either be inherited or may appear over a period of time due to some genetic mutations. For instance, even if a person is born with a normal

51

heart, he can develop severe heart conditions over time because of environmental conditions like his lifestyle. The normal genetic code that determines the functioning of the heart is altered leading to an abnormality.

As for Restless Leg Syndrome, the most common environmental factor is iron deficiency. Now this low iron level may occur during pregnancy, just after birth, during childhood or well into adulthood. The first probability with respect to genetics is that the iron levels cause small changes in certain genes. These changes are powerful enough to lead to a chain of conditions that progress into RLS symptoms. One gene that has been observed in great detail is a gene called BTDB9. In almost 75% of individuals who suffer from RLS, this gene is considered to be responsible. A small variation in this gene is responsible for the development of RLS.

Studies have revealed that the interaction between this gene and iron regulation does exist. It was this understanding that made it possible to link our genes to iron deficiency as a trigger to set off Restless Leg Syndrome.

The first person to postulate the possibility of the influence of genetics in RLS was Ekbom, after whom the condition is partially named. He suggested that people with RLS most often inherit the condition form their immediate family or their relatives. This theory was based on several case studies that showed up to 5 generations in a family who had inherited the condition.

In the year 1960, familial aggregation was also described for this condition. Familial aggregation means that a cluster of similar conditions can be seen in a family, making the probability of inheriting these conditions higher. This is usually the first step towards determining hereditary causes for a certain disease. Once the cluster has been observed, it is easier to provide a hypothesis based on the genes that are affected.

The studies revealed that RLS shows a dominant autosomal inheritance pattern. This means that the person affected usually has one biological parent who suffers from the condition. Also, the sibling of the person might be affected. However, it is not possible to rule out the chance that one may inherit the condition from other relatives. But, most studies show that the parent is usually affected. Especially when you consider cases of early onset of Restless Leg Syndrome, the condition is usually passed on by the parent.

In the year 2000, the genetic variation for RLS was noted to be phenotypic. Phenotypic variations are the root cause of evolution. It is these variations that are passed on from one generation to the other, sometimes continuously. To understand this better, a study was conducted on monozygotic twins. Out of the 12 pairs of twins who were used in the study, 10 of them were diagnosed with definite Restless Leg Syndrome. This study, conducted by the International Restless Leg Syndrome Study Group revealed that although the rate of inheritance was high, the description of the symptoms and the probable age of onset varied drastically.

A clinical review on RLS management was presented in the year 2003 by Earley. His studies showed that the association with familial history was maximum in female patients who showed an early onset of the symptoms.

It is currently proposed that the 12q chromosome is responsible for the susceptibility to Restless Leg Syndrome. Of course, there are also several other loci that may also be mapped to understand this condition better.

You see, the basic function of several genes in our brain, not just with respect to RLS, is also under a lot of scrutiny by the scientific community. It is impossible to exactly determine how our genes control our brain, allowing it to perform so many complex functions at one given time.

The only important thing is to understand what the triggers for these mutations are. As for RLS, most of the studies associating genetics with the condition are centred around iron deficiency. The debate currently is whether it is the iron deficiency which is causing the mutation. Another possibility is that the genes are changing as a response to this low iron level.

It is important to understand whether the proteins responsible for iron management have anything to do with the proteins that are present in the genes that have been mapped for RLS. Alternatively, we could also consider the proteins associated with dopamine. It is probably these proteins that are responsible for iron management, and consecutively our genes.

The only evidence we have to genetic role in RLS is the inheritance pattern of the condition. However, when the exact loci for the condition can be located, there could be unbelievable breakthroughs in the treatment of this condition. It will be possible not only to find a more definite approach to treatment but also control the condition from the fatal level. That is when we will be successful at controlling the prevalence of the condition in a given population.

3. The Role of Nutrients

Iron

One of the most researched and well known causes of Restless Leg Syndrome is iron deficiency. The first person to recognise the possibility of such an association was Professor Nor lander. He reported that when patients were treated for iron deficiency, they showed notable improvements in the symptoms. In some cases, the condition was completely eliminated.

There is a very strong connection between vitamin deficiency and RLS. However, the occurrence of iron deficiency in patients with RLS is less. What I mean is that only 15% of the population that is affected with RLS shows any significant iron deficiency. So, the only possible explanation for this is that the serum iron levels are normal while there is an iron deficiency in the tissues. To evaluate this theory postulated by Professor Norlander, several studies were conducted on the brain tissues.

All the studies available till date support the fact that an iron deficiency, in fact, does exist in the brain of patients with RLS. This is despite the fact that their blood tests reveal normal iron levels. The spinal sap has been extracted using a procedure called a lumbar puncture to further study the connection of iron with RLS. This process involves obtaining the cerebrospinal fluid from the lower region of the spine with a huge needle. This fluid contains all the chemicals and the proteins that are present inside the brain. This fluid has revealed that the protein responsible for iron storage, ferritin, is very low in count. So, even if the patients are not really anaemic with normal iron levels in the serum, they show RLS symptoms.

Several MRI scans have also revealed that the iron concentration in the brain is extremely low with patients who have RLS. Now these iron levels are noticeably low in the substantia nigra region which is also responsible for dopamine production. This is how another connection between dopamine and RLS can be made.

To study the relationship between iron deficiency and RLS, a special brain bank has been set up by the RLS foundation. This brain bank stores tissues of the brains of individuals who have RLS and have agreed to donate their brains for medical research after death. These tissues have strengthened the belief that the reduction in the number of iron receptors is the core of the relationship between iron and RLS.

Although there is enough research on peripheral iron synthesis, we are still quite unaware of the barrier between the brain and blood iron levels. The next question to answer would be how the brain cells can have iron deficiency while all the other organs in the body have normal iron levels? This is quite puzzling as iron deficiency is one of the most definite causes of RLS.

Magnesium

If you are someone who is not really fond of healthy foods like nuts, grains and leafy veggies, you might want to reconsider your diet. It is these foods that provide the richest source of magnesium, one of the most important minerals for our body. It is so important because every organ, including the heart, kidney and the skeletal system need magnesium to function normally. The main functions of magnesium in the body are regulation of calcium and enzyme production.

True magnesium deficiency rarely occurs in people. However, there are several conditions like diabetes and pancreatitis that can cause an imbalance in the magnesium levels in the body. RLS and sleeplessness are among the most common symptoms of magnesium deficiency.

According to the US department of Agriculture, it was observed that magnesium is one of the most important factors in iron regulation. It was observed that people who display long term insomnia or unconventional brain waves when they are asleep usually had magnesium deficiency. The study was first conducted on 12 elderly subjects. When they were given magnesium, they were able to fall asleep easily. A similar result was obtained when the experiment was conducted on a group of subjects who were alcoholic.

Doctors who practice holistic medicine, especially, will tell you that magnesium therapy is one of the best ways to relieve RLS symptoms. According to the Nutritional Magnesium Association, magnesium has the ability to relax our nerves and muscles. While calcium contracts the muscle fibres, magnesium relaxes them. So, if you have more calcium and less magnesium in the body, you can feel various forms of muscle contraction including convulsions, twitches and even jerks.

The role of magnesium is to regulate the amount of calcium that enters the neurons. A small amount of calcium is necessary for the brain to transmit information in the form of mild electrical signals. Magnesium lets the calcium in just long enough for the signal to be transmitted and then forces it back. If there is too much calcium in the brain, the delicate neurons become extremely irritated. When the neurons are irritated, they tend to pass signals repeatedly. This consumes a lot of energy, eventually leading to the death of the cell.

This over activity of the neurons also results in constant contraction of the muscles. This explains all the symptoms that one experiences with RLS including the soreness of the muscles, muscle spasms, cramps and also muscle fatigue. The tingling sensations and the unpleasant feelings in the legs that cause the urge to move the limb might be due to magnesium deficiency.

For several individuals with RLS, enriching their diet with foods that are rich in magnesium has brought a lot of relief from the symptoms. Using magnesium supplements have also proved to be quite helpful in controlling the symptoms if not eliminating them completely. The relaxing quality of magnesium is one of the most important factors in treating RLS.

Vitamins

There are three important vitamins that are responsible for the symptoms of RLS. These vitamins include Vitamin D, Vitamin B12 and Vitamin E. Studies have revealed that treatment with these vitamins have provided positive results with the RLS symptoms.

Vitamin B12

This is probably the most important vitamin as far as RLS symptoms go. Deficiency of vitamin B12 can cause RLS in 2 ways.

First, when the body is deprived of Vitamin B12, a lot of damage is caused in the central nervous system. This damage also includes the brain. The damage caused by Vitamin B12 deficiency can also extend to other parts of the brain that are responsible for the motor commands given to the rest of the body.

Restless Leg Syndrome is mostly related to poor coordination in the limbs. When the movements are not controlled or inhibited effectively, the symptoms of RLS appear. A drop in the level of

Vitamin B12 in our body may be responsible for this as the neurons that are responsible for the motor functions are also damaged.

The damage that I talk about here does not necessarily imply that the cells in the brain are physically damaged. It does not refer to cell death either. Sometimes, the enzymes that are produced to enable these neurons to transmit messages may become dysfunctional. There are several proteins that come to the surface in the region of the nervous system called the substantia nigra. These proteins prevent the absorption of Iron, leading to the symptoms of RLS.

Like we saw in the previous section, a low level of iron in the Cerebrospinal Fluid is one of the clearest indicators for RLS. In fact, when a person is anaemic, he experiences the loss of both iron and Vitamin B12 which results in severe restless leg symptoms. It is a common thing to provide vitamin B12 supplementation for people who have anaemia. This is a clear indication that Vitamin B12 has an important role to play in the regulation of iron in our body.

Of course, there is no direct link available to support the connection between Vitamin B12 and Restless Leg Syndrome. In most people the deficiency of Vitamin B12 goes undetected. But, whenever iron deficiency is recorded, Vitamin B12 becomes a part of the treatment process.

In the year 1993, as study conducted to evaluate the relationship between Vitamin B12 and RLS was published in the Journal of Postgraduate Medicine. This test was conducted on elderly patients with RLS. It was noted that Vitamin B12 and iron deficiencies were most common among these patients. These two deficiencies were also more easily treatable that other causal factors of RLS. In patients who had severe B12 deficiency a marked relief from the symptoms was observed in the very first month of treatment using Vitamin B12 supplements.

Another study conducted by the New York University suggests that although B12 supplements do not directly result in relief from symptoms of RLS, they act as a support system for our RBCs and also the nervous system, leading to relief from symptoms.

Vitamin D

A recent study published in the Neuropsychiatric disease and Treatment revealed that Vitamin D deficiency could be one of the most important causal factors in Restless Leg Syndrome.

This condition develops primarily due to neurological dysfunction. Now, vitamin D, which is also known as the sunshine vitamin, plays a vital role in regulating the function of the nervous system. So, it is quite natural that this vitamin is also responsible for RLS. This connection between RLS and vitamin E has been proposed by several researchers. However, there are few studies available to actually support this hypothesis.

One of the most recent studies to connect the two was conducted on a test group of 155 individuals. The level of Vitamin D in these patients were analysed and they were divided into two groups. The first group consisted of members who had vitamin D deficiency and the second group consisted of members who did not have vitamin deficiency.

The research on these two groups suggested that 50% of the individuals with vitamin D deficiency also had RLS while only 6.8% of individuals without Vitamin D deficiency had RLS. These results showed that deficiency of Vitamin D increased the prevalence of this condition.

The symptoms suggested by the International RLS Rating scale were seen in those who had Vitamin D deficiency. These results were based on a questionnaire that was used to understand the symptoms experienced by the members of this study group.

Vitamin D has also been linked to sleep disorders, making it a high suspect in RLS as well. When we fall asleep, we reach a state called Rapid Eye Movement or REM sleep. That is when we tend to dream. Now, when REM is disrupted, several sleep disorders arise. These disruptions could be in the form of several hormone fluctuations and also RLS which leads to uncontrollable limb movement at night.

In the journal "Medical Hypothesis", a clinical trial was published to elucidate this relationship between Vitamin D and insomnia. The study was conducted on a group of 1500 patients over 2 years. During the course of this study a steady Vitamin D3 level was maintained in these patients. Now, many of these patients had a history of various sleep disorders. When the vitamin D3 level was kept normal, they did not show the symptoms of any sleep disorder and were able to fall asleep normally.

There are also several studies related to sleeplessness in children. A recent study was conducted in the year 2014. The study was titled, "the effect of Vitamin D Supplements of Severity of RLS". The study followed a group of 12 individuals. All of them were diagnosed with primary RLS along with Vitamin D deficiency. When they were given Vitamin D supplements and when the levels were resorted to normal, the severity of the symptoms of RLS also reduced considerably.

There are many such studies that are available to correlate Vitamin D to RLS and several other sleep disorders.

Vitamin E

The main role of Vitamin E is to protect the tissues in the body. It is an antioxidant which keeps the cells protected. Sometimes when the fat absorption is affected or when a person is born underweight, then there is a Vitamin E deficiency in the body. Any other problem in your fat metabolism can lead to Vitamin E deficiency.

While the most common issues of Vitamin E are related to dermatological studies, the effect of this nutrient on the brain is often overlooked. It is this effect on the brain that can also lead to RLS symptoms.

The primary function of Vitamin E with respect to the brain is protection of the brain cells. This fact has been elucidated through studies conducted on individuals who are suffering from Alzheimer's and Dementia. A study conducted on 341 patients who were treated with Vitamin E revealed that the progression of Alzheimer's was delayed. Even after diagnosis of the condition, it was seen that the deterioration of the individual's ability to carry out daily activities was considerably delayed when effective Vitamin E treatment was provided.

Another article published in the 2004 edition of The New England Journal Medicine revealed that Vitamin E can also reduce the progression of diseases like dementia. While these studies are interesting, the next thing we need to understand is how this nutrient can cause RLS.

First, the brain cells are protected by Vitamin E, preventing issues like reduced dopamine receptors that have been connected to RLS symptoms. The transmission of nerve impulses is also regulated by Vitamin E. When the impulses are not passed on properly, the neurotransmitters are produced excessively. This causes symptoms that resemble RLS.

There are also various tendon reflexes that are caused when Vitamin E levels are low. Muscular fatigue is also common in case of Vitamin E deficiency. Most neurological complications can be solved with Vitamin E deficiency.

Clinical investigations have revealed that individuals who suffer from terrible nocturnal cramps have been relieved of the symptoms when they are treated with Vitamin E. These positive results were also observed in smaller groups with participants who had RLS.

There is another hypothesis with respect to the relationship between RLS and Vitamin E deficiency. When this antioxidant level drops, there are several free radicals in the body. These free radicals are highly reactive molecules that tend to oxidise the cells. This leads to oxidative damage of the cells. Similarly, even the red blood cells are damaged. The main component of the RBCs is iron. The name haemoglobin itself means iron and protein. When these cells are damaged, the iron level falls making the person anaemic.

We know now that iron is one of the most important nutrients required to prevent RLS symptoms. Although it is not known if Vitamin E deficiency is directly linked to RLS or not, the studies conducted until most recently have shown that Vitamin E treatment can provide significant relief from the symptoms of the condition.

Food Allergies

There are some food allergies that can act as triggers for RLS symptoms. One of the most common foods allergies observed in RLS patients is gluten allergy. When a person is allergic to any food item, the symptoms are seen immediately. However, sometimes, the changes can be very subtle and long term. Gluten allergy, for instance, can change the way your body absorbs nutrients. This can lead to vitamin deficiencies that eventually affect blood circulation and your nervous system. Thus, RLS symptoms can be triggered due to food allergies. There are various types of allergies that can be held responsible. So, if you know of any foods that you are allergic to, make sure you tell your doctor about it for proper diagnosis.

4. The Role of Medicines

Antidepressants

There have been several clinical investigations about the effects of antidepressants on RLS symptoms. The observations made by doctors and researchers have shown that the symptoms increase when a person is taking any antipsychotic or antidepressant medication.

In one of these clinical studies, the observations were based on individuals who were given antidepressants for the first time. The purpose of this study was to check if RLS is caused due to these antidepressants or whether the symptoms are worsened due to this condition. It was observed that 9% of the patients in this test group developed RLS as a side effect to the antidepressants. In about 28% of the patients, the symptoms were provoked as a result of these antidepressants. A variety of antidepressants were given to the individuals who participated in this test. While some of them shown immediate fluctuations in the RLS symptoms, others had no effect at all. In a small percentage, the symptoms also deteriorated.

With this test it was confirmed that antidepressants have an effect on RLS. The theory behind the effect of antidepressants leads us to the neurotransmitter serotonin. Most of these antidepressants act as serotonin inhibitors causing a disturbance in the sleep cycle. These disturbances are also extended to the production of dopamine as the two neurotransmitters are meant to balance one another. When one of them goes off balance, the other one naturally falls off balance.

People who are on antidepressants are also psychologically affected. This strengthens the symptoms making it hard for them to cope with RLS.

Antihistamines

Antihistamines are basically medicines that are taken to prevent allergies of any sort. These medicines are useful in blocking reception of histamines. Now, there are two types of histamine receptors in our body, H1 and H2. When H1 is stimulated, we tend to have reactions like itching, rashes etc. These antihistamines may either reduce the reception of histamine or may reduce the number of receptors present.

Either way, they are used to treat a number of allergies including hay fever, pet allergies, cold, food allergies and even a regular cold. If you have seasonal allergies, you must be familiar with the use of antihistamine medicines.

Sometimes, the side effect of this drug is in the form of RLS symptoms. You may either develop these symptoms with regular use of the drugs or if you have existing RLS symptoms, they will simply aggravate with the use of antihistamines.

These side effects arise because antihistamines may also block the dopamine receptors in the brain. So, the signals that are transmitted from one neuron to another are not transmitted properly, making it necessary for the body to produce excessive dopamine. As you know, this may cause RLS symptoms as the sleep cycle is severely affected. So, if you already have RLS symptoms, you must make sure you mention this to the doctor who is treating you. Usually, a type of antihistamines called "Secondary antihistamines" may not cause such severe RLS symptoms or may not cause them at all.

Over the counter drugs

There are many over the counter medicines that are prescribed as a remedy for RLS. Usually, these medicines include pain relievers such as acetaminophen. There are also several anti-inflammatory drugs that are known to relieve the symptoms of RLS. These medicines include Naproxen, Ibuprofen and Ketoprofen. These medicines are non-steroidal and seldom have any effect on the neurotransmitters or on the hormones and enzymes produced in the body.

However, even with these medicines, excessive consumption can aggravate the symptoms of RLS. There are several other over the counter medicines that we take for flu and other common ailments that can cause RLS symptoms as a side effect.

If you are already suffering from RLS, you must be attentive to all the reactions caused by certain medicines. If you are taking some medicine for the first time and you have never had RLS before, then there are chances that it is that medicine that is causing these symptoms.

You may contact your doctor when you experience such symptoms. By reducing the dosage of the medicine or by using an alternative, you should be able to relieve yourself of the common symptoms of Restless Leg Syndrome.

Sometimes, these medicines may block receptors of several neurotransmitters, causing the symptoms to appear or aggravate. While the exact mechanism of these medicines is not entirely known, you must always avoid over the counter medicines without consulting a doctor, especially when you have RLS. Any possibility of increased symptoms must be avoided altogether.

Anti-Nausea Medication

Anti-nausea medicines are also known as antiemetic medicines. These medicines are able to prevent vomiting, nausea and related digestive problems. Commonly, these medicines do not have any side effects. However, in case of individuals who have been diagnosed with possible, probable or even definite RLS, the medicines that they consume must be scrutinised to a large extent. It is possible that the symptoms are aggravated when you take any medicine.

Generally, the anti-nausea medicines that cause RLS symptoms include Dramamine, Phenegran, Reglan and Comapzine. I know these names from personal experience and also through the testimonies of other individuals I know with the condition.

There are some alternative drugs that may not make the symptoms of RLS worse. These medicines are usually given for motion sickness. The common ones are Zofran and Transderm Scop. They are probably milder and have a different mechanism in the body, making them safe to consume.

However, with the drugs that do cause RLS symptoms, their reaction in the body is very similar to the anti-histamine medication. They tend to block the dopamine receptors in the brain, causing a chain of reactions that lead to symptoms similar to RLS. These medicines are called dopamine receptor antagonists and have an action exactly opposite to the dopamine receptor agonists which are used in treating RLS.

When you notice the symptoms increasing or even beginning, make sure you reduce the dosage or stop consuming the medicine. If this doesn't help, then the trigger may be something else.

5. The Role of Pregnancy

During pregnancy RLS is very common. More than two thirds of expecting mothers show RLS symptoms. It is possible that these symptoms begin during pregnancy and are only observed during the pregnancy. On the other hand, women who have mild or probable RLS may develop severe symptoms during their pregnancy.

In a study conducted in Italy, it was observed that out of 600 women who participated in the study, 161 of them showed RLS symptoms during their pregnancy. That was about 27% of the whole study group. In this study group, 60% of them had experienced RLS symptoms before. Out of this group some of them, precisely 11%, showed an improvement in the symptoms. For 28% of them, the symptoms remained the same. For the remaining members of the group, after the onset of pregnancy, the symptoms became severe, especially towards their third trimester.

For most of these women, the symptoms decreased to a great extent after delivery. For only 8 women, the symptoms remained for close to 6 months post-delivery. A follow up study was conducted with 207 pregnant women. Out of them, 73 already had RLS symptoms. It was noted that RLS symptoms became terrible with women who had transient RLS showed an increased risk of severe symptoms. On the other hand, the women who did not have RLS during pregnancy were safer in comparison.

Similar studies conducted across the world have had three similar outcomes:

- The condition is extremely prevalent among women, affecting close to 1 in every 5 pregnant women.

- For most of these women, the condition lasts only until delivery and is either completely resolved or significantly reduced.

- The symptoms become severe towards the third trimester.

During pregnancy, it becomes extremely difficult to differentiate between the symptoms or RLS and the leg cramps that are quite common during this period. This condition can also lead to sleep disturbances and fatigue. The biggest differentiator between RLS symptoms and leg cramps is that the former appears in spurts while the latter is very painful and is quite prolonged. In case of cramps, the muscles become extremely hardened and are contracted leading to extreme pain.

There are several reasons for RLS symptoms during pregnancy. There are four main reasons for developing RLS symptoms during pregnancy. They are:
- A history of the condition in the family. For women with familial history, the chances of developing RLS during pregnancy are 8 times.
- A history of RLS before pregnancy. For women who have had RLS just before pregnancy, the chances of developing the symptoms are 5 times.
- A history of RLS at any time in their life. For these women, the risk of developing the condition is 13 times.
- Low RBC count leading to reduced iron levels. For these women, the risk of developing the condition is doubled.

Usually RLS symptoms during pregnancy are transient. This means that the symptoms only occur for the period of pregnancy.

However, if a women does develop transient RLS, she is at a high risk of developing a severe condition in the future in comparison to a woman who has not experienced RLS symptoms during pregnancy.

While research suggests RLS symptoms in pregnant women as a genetic predisposition, there is no delineated explanation for the causes of RLS or the increased symptoms during pregnancy. In fact there are so many possibilities with respect to RLS and pregnancy that it is difficult to point out to one specific causal factor. For instance, low minerals and vitamins, the reduced capacity of the bladder, varicose veins, nerve compression, hormonal changes and even oedema could be responsible for RLS symptoms becoming severe during pregnancy.

Since there is no evidence to support the exact causal symptoms of RLS during pregnancy, very little is also known about the possible treatments for this condition during pregnancy. There are a few medicines that have been extremely useful in controlling the symptoms and providing some relief.

However, there is no medication that has been approved by the FDA till date. Usually, women who experience the symptoms of RLS before pregnancy are advised to stop consuming these medicines when they are pregnant. The only available reference is the rating provided by FDA. These medications are classified as A, B, C, D and X. Drugs marked A pose the least risk while the ones classified as X should be avoided.

No matter what treatment you start or continue during pregnancy, you must always consult your physician. You must take into account several factors like the effect it has on the baby, the effects on breastfeeding etc. It is always recommended that unless it is vital, medication for RLS should be avoided during pregnancy. The benefits provided by the medicine must outweigh the possible risks if you want to consume the medicine.

There are several prenatal vitamins that you may consume during your pregnancy. You may also require iron supplements. These dietary supplements are considered safe and are known to have positive results on the symptoms of RLS. Since anaemia and iron deficiency are the primary contributors to the symptoms of RLS, you can control the symptoms to a large extent when you take safe and recommended supplements.

6. RLS as a Secondary Condition

Many times, an existing medical condition may lead to RLS symptoms. You must make sure you tell your doctor about all the medical conditions that you have been diagnosed for in the past. You must also insist on having these conditions investigated to make sure you get the right treatment. There are several primary conditions that you need to pay attention to with respect to RLS as a secondary symptom. Here are some medical conditions that can cause RLS.

Chronic Kidney Disease or Other Kidney Problems

When a person has Chronic Kidney Disease, the first symptom is a drastic reduction in the iron level leading to RLS symptoms. When your kidneys are healthy, they produce a hormone called erythropoietin. This hormone is responsible for the production of our Red Blood Cells. When the kidneys are damaged for any reason, the level of this hormone drops as well. Also, when the iron available in the body is less, the number of healthy red blood cells also reduces. Usually, this reduction in the RBC count is noticed in the early stages of renal problems itself. It gets worse with progression of the condition. It has been noticed that any patient who is in the last stage of a renal disease always has anaemia.

Another cause for RLS during renal failure is the reduced level of the Parathyroid Hormone. This hormone acts as a calcium regulator and is hence important in enabling neural transmissions. When a person is diagnosed with any kidney condition, there is a high chance that he or she may develop some bone disease.

Therefore, doctors always check the levels of the Parathyroid Hormone in the individual.

In order to control renal problems, several psychiatric and neurological drugs are also administered. This leads to low PTH that lead to symptoms of RLS.

The only possible treatment in chronic kidney failure or in end stage renal diseases is dialysis. This has a very big implication for individuals who already have RLS or for those who have developed RLS due to renal failure.

The main purpose of dialysis is to act as a replacement for the kidney function which is lost due to a renal disease. There are two main types of dialysis, namely peritoneal dialysis and hemodialysis. Both types of dialysis may have the same implications for an individual suffering from RLS.

For over 40 years, the effects of dialysis on RLS have been studied in great detail. It has been noticed that RLS is a common problem with individuals who have and End Stage Renal Disease, both before and after dialysis. According to these studies 33% of individuals with End Stage Renal Disease will develop RLS eventually. They experience periodic limb movements as an individual condition or in association with RLS. 70% of individuals who experience periodic limb movements will develop RLS as well.

There are several other factors that lead to RLS in individuals with renal problems. This includes age, the gender, the possibility of diabetes as well etc. Even body weight can cause RLS when you have a renal disease.

For patients who are undergoing dialysis, they need to be screened for RLS in the beginning because the incidence is extremely high. With dialysis comes an increased loss of iron. This causes increased symptoms of Restless Leg Syndrome which may become hard to manage eventually.

When RLS becomes extremely severe, it also means that the individual will not be able to move as freely as before. The cramps and the muscle contractions can restrict movement, making the period of dialysis harder on the person. Even the process of dialysis is hard as the person has to sit in one place for close to three hours. This may trigger off symptoms of RLS as well. This challenge also extends to the caretakers of the person as they have to deal with the constant urge to move the feet and the need to remain in once place in case of kidney failure.

According to a recent study, it was noticed that the discomfort in the limbs were stimulated by the reclining position assumed by a person when he is undergoing dialysis. Of course, dialysis cannot be ruled out in this stage of renal failure. There may be some non-medicinal options that one can opt for to get some comfort from this condition.

Therefore, the type of dialysis and the timing of the procedure should be customised to each individual, especially when he or she has been diagnosed with definite restless leg syndrome.

Diabetes

With diabetes, especially Type 2 diabetes, there is a slow deterioration of nerves, making you more sensitive to sensations such as pain. The causes for this type of nerve damage vary from one individual to another. However, the most common cause for the damage is having high blood sugar for a long period of time.

Peripheral neuropathy is one of the most common issues when it comes to diabetic nerve damage. This mostly affects the legs and the feet, leading to several foot problems including a loss in sensations in your feet. If you have ever noticed how people with diabetes are advised to ensure that they have no foot injuries, this neuropathy is the reason for that. Since there is no sensation in the feet, any sore or cut can go unnoticed and lead to severe infection. This type of neuropathy very rarely affects other body parts such as the back, the abdomen and the arms. If you can connect this to RLS, you will also realise that RLS symptoms are commonly seen in these body parts. When there is peripheral neuropathy, the following symptoms are noticed:

- Tingling of the feet
- Burning sensations
- Pain
- Numbness

These symptoms aggravate in the evenings, just as they do in case of Restless Leg Syndrome. Studies also show that RLS is highly associated with diabetes. Research conducted in Italy on 124 patients with diabetes and a control group of 87 individuals proved that there is a connection between the two conditions. The results revealed that 18% of the individuals with diabetes had Restless Leg Syndrome in comparison to the 5.5% of individuals in the control group.

The studies were conducted with multiple variables. This also showed that the symptoms of RLS depended on various other factors like the BMI, age and gender of the individual. The presence of neuropathy was another important condition for the development of RLS symptoms.

With RLS and diabetes, there are several other conditions that tend to worsen the symptoms. When the symptoms of RLS increase, sleep quality deteriorates. Additionally, even falling asleep and staying asleep becomes difficult. With chronic sleep disorders, there is also a high risk of developing cardiovascular problems. It may also be fatal in case of individuals who have severe diabetes.

It is because of this progression that RLS is commonly associated with heart diseases as well. Most often, a person will have RLS related heart problems when he also suffers from diabetes. The sleep disorder also makes it hard to manage diabetes. The health effects when you have both RLS and diabetes are long term.

According to one recent study conducted on 121 patients out of whom 54 had definite RLS, the prevalence of RLS among people with diabetes was confirmed. In addition to this, it was also observed that insulin and other oral medicines that were taken to provide relief from diabetes were capable of aggravating the symptoms. So, the primary concern with many doctors is to help individuals with RLS manage their sugar levels.

Peripheral Neuropathy

A neuropathy is a condition of the nervous system which leads to burning, painful and shooting sensations in the legs and the arms. There are various causes like diabetes, HIV infection, Vitamin Deficiencies, alcoholism and also rheumatoid arthritis that can lead to peripheral neuropathy. However, one of the most common causes of peripheral neuropathy is mechanical compression. When the nerve is damaged due to stress, trauma, accident or any injury, neuropathy may occur. Compression of the nerves in the thigh nerves leads to a condition called Meralgia Paresthetica which is quite an uncommon condition. There are severe burning sensations and tingling sensations on the frontal region of the thigh as well as the sides. This problem occurs between the age of 30 to 60 years. It may go away by itself or may require medical attention. Any compression of the nervous system leads to sensations that are quite characteristic of RLS.

Tarsal Tunnel Syndrome

A certain nerve called the tibial nerve runs down the leg until the ankle. It is a branch of the primary nerve that comes down to the legs. When there is a compression in this nerve due to aging, accidents or any sort of injury, tarsal tunnel syndrome occurs. These injuries lead to inflammation near the ankle which leads to a tingling and burning sensation. It is very similar to an electric shock. These symptoms are usually felt near the ankle and at the bottom of the feet. Sometimes, the pain can be isolated and may occur either in the arch of the foot, the toes and the calf region.

These symptoms can also be caused when a person is flat footed or has some abnormality in his nerve such as a ganglion cyst, bone spurs, inflammations and swollen tendons etc. They can also manifest as secondary symptoms of conditions like arthritis or diabetes. Since these symptoms and associated conditions are common to RLS, there are several speculations that the condition is caused by tarsal tunnel syndrome. Experiments conducted on middle aged subjects with a year or more of tarsal tunnel symptoms revealed that painful leg and toe movements were caused by the neuropathies.

Rheumatoid Arthritis

RLS is partly considered a disease related to the nervous system. This condition interplays with sleep and immunity. Another common condition that is seen when a person is diagnosed with Rheumatoid Arthritis is iron deficiency; the biggest contributor to RLS. However, Rheumatoid arthritis is caused by chronic inflammation caused by cytokines. There are various immunomodulatory alterations that are noticed when a person has Rheumatoid Arthritis. These changes are responsible for all the sleep disorders that occur, including RLS. In a study conducted almost 3 decades ago, it was noticed that 30% of the patients with Rheumatoid Arthritis also showed symptoms of RLS. Even the recent studies conducted have shown similar results. It has been observed that RLS is quite common in most patients with other connective tissue disorders like scleroderma, Sjoren's syndrome etc.

Circulatory Problems

Cramping of the legs or various parts of the body is usually caused by circulatory issues. Many RLS symptoms can be reduced when appropriate treatment is given to improve circulation of blood in the affected part of the body. Although there is no clinical study available to elucidate this speculation, the results shown by the treatment gives enough reason to believe that RLS is a result of improper circulation.

One specific circulatory condition that is related to RLS is erythromelaglia which is a type of peripheral neuropathy. This is a neurovascular condition where the blood vessels in the hands and legs are blocked on and off. This leads to severe burning sensations and pain in the affected area. The symptoms are aggravated with sleep disorders. So, it is believed that the conditions are interrelated as the symptoms and the causal factors are interrelated.

Reflex Sympathetic Dystrophy

RLS is also associated with Reflex sympathetic dystrophy. This is a condition caused by the irritation of the nervous system. Any abnormal excitement of the nervous system triggers impulses that are very similar to RLS. Burning and tingling sensations in the arms and the legs along with tenderness of the skin is common in case of reflex sympathetic dystrophy.

Like RLS, this condition also does not have a clear causal factor. However, it is certain that the peripheral nervous system and the brain have an important role to play in this condition. It is possible that RLS occurs as a secondary condition when a person has reflex sympathetic dystrophy as the peripheral nervous system is affected.

Metatarsalgia and Morton's Neuroma

With this condition, the ball of the foot becomes inflamed. This leads to painful sensations that shoot up the leg. Usually, this condition is caused by wearing poorly fitting shoes or by carrying out activities like running or skipping that put pressure on the foot. The sensations include a sharp shooting pain in the leg along with burning sensations.

Metatarsalgia is related to another condition called Morton's neuroma. In this condition, there are certain non-cancerous growths that occur near the head of your third and fourth metatarsal heads. This is also a condition that is caused by stress on the feet with improper footwear or intense activity.

An intensive study to check for any association between these conditions and RLS was conducted on a 42 year old woman. She had been diagnosed with several neuromas in both the feet. Repeated neuroma injections and treatment methods were used to excise these neuromas. It was observed that the restlessness in the feet was reduced by about 85%. Sleep was better and the periodic limb movements reduced as well. These neuromas also cause foot dysesthesias which lead to RLS symptoms.

Liver Failure

RLS symptoms are seen in 16% of people with liver cirrhosis. The association between liver failure or chronic liver problems is not supported by many studies. Some studies have been published. One such study was carried out in King Abdulaziz Medical City, King Fahad National Guard Hospital and King Khalid University Hospital. The data was collected after studying 201 patients with confirmed liver cirrhosis. The data was obtained using an RLS questionnaire. Although there was no association observed between the severity of the liver problem and RLS, it was confirmed that RLS is very common among patients with RLS.

Obesity

Being obese or overweight can increase the risk of developing RLS symptoms. A study published in the April edition of the Medical Journal of the American Academy of Neurology, 'Neurology' showed that overweight people were at 60% higher risk of developing the condition. It is possible that the eating habits and the associated dopamine levels cause increased RLS symptoms.

Two large studies at the Nurses' Health Study and the Health Professional Follow Up Study, it was observed the prevalence of

RLS symptoms in 6.5% of the female subjects and 4.1% of the male subjects increased with an increase in the circumference of the waist and the increased body mass index suggesting that obesity could be a cause for RLS. This also affects the sleeping patterns, leading to increased RLS symptoms.

Allergy to certain foods

Some people I spoke to in forums were convinced that they were allergic to some foods. If you think this applies to you, ask your doctor for an allergy test.

7. Can RLS be Psychosomatic?

For a very long time, I used to get really offended with the "It's all in the mind" statement that people use when you talk to them about a condition you are suffering from. But, my research helped me realise that for some people these symptoms could actually be associated with their mind. The name psychosomatic talks about two things, the physical level of the condition and the mental level of any condition.

It has been observed that some conditions like Restless Leg Syndrome can become worse when there is an underlying mental condition as well. You see, all the physical conditions that we are aware of have their own methods of treatment. However, with psychosomatic conditions, you also need to extend the treatment to the social and mental layers of an individual. Since the physical being and the mental being are exclusive and still so interdependent, you might see this as a rather difficult challenge.

When you are under stress or are experiencing any type of emotional stress, your body undergoes a series of changes. The most common ones include:

- Dryness in the mouth
- Sweating
- Heart Palpitations

- Tremors
- Chest Pain
- Fast breathing
- Headaches
- Nausea

It is also believed that Restless Leg Syndrome is an after effect of any sort of mental trauma or stress. When this was first suspected, several studies were conducted to determine whether this ailment could actually be psychosomatic.

A very popular study was conducted on 100 patients who were newly diagnosed with RLS. These patients were categories as mild or severe depending upon the type of symptoms they experienced. The symptoms were rated as per the standards of the International RLS study group.

The participants of this study were made to fill out the Pittsburgh Sleep Quality Index along with other tests to check their quality of sleep. They also had to answer a simple questionnaire that evaluated their symptoms. The test scores and demographics were collected to facilitate this study. There was also a control group that consisted of 37 participants.

The studies revealed that most of the patients with RLS also had comorbid psychosomatic symptoms. This was an important contributing factor for all the symptoms of RLS. It was observed that when the symptoms were severe, the chances of the psychosomatic domain were much higher.

One of the largest individual contributing factors to this type of somatization of the symptoms was anxiety. Since the patients with severe RLS also had extreme sleep deprivation, it was observed that anxiety was also on the rise. The question is which condition is influenced by the other?

Anxiety and stress have been known to play a very important role in Restless Leg Syndrome. From one of the testimonies that I heard recently, the symptoms can get so bad that you will actually feel a pounding sensation in your years. Some of them who suffer from anxiety are unable to sleep well due to their stress. This is an added reason for them to feel uneasy and fatigued. I have read about people going for as long as 48 hours without sleeping. The sad part is even when you are extremely exhausted and sleep deprived, you cannot fall asleep!

The whole cycle of anxiety, stress and RLS is quite vicious. One factor aggravates the other. What I mean is that when you are very stressed, your RLS symptoms get worse. Then, because you are unable to fall asleep, you wake up feeling even more stressed out.

For me, whenever I am stressed at work or even have the slightest emotional distress I have a constant uneasy feeling at the pit of my stomach. This is because I know that I am not going to get enough sleep. This feeling is common among many individuals with RLS. It is the same feeling you have when you are in a plane and you dread the taking off and the landing bit!

Dopamine also has a very important role to play in stress management. Under regular conditions, stress is described as a condition when you see some threat to your safety. This is momentary and requires you to react instantly. This is called the flight or fight mechanism. Now, the body has a great stress management system that is equipped to respond when you feel momentary tension and stress. Dopamine is released to help you cope with a stressful condition.

However, if the stress is prolonged, for example a very demanding job, the response mechanism becomes unstable. The dopamine levels can go haywire in the body, leading to RLS symptoms. Especially in people who already have RLS, stress can aggravate the symptoms of RLS to a large extent.

Lastly when you have been diagnosed with clinical depression, anxiety disorder or stress, medication becomes necessary. This includes antidepressants. We have already learnt in the previous section that antidepressants act as dopamine blockers, causing an increase in the RLS symptoms. So, you see, the psyche also has an important role to play in regulating the response of your central nervous system. With a condition like RLS especially, the symptoms and the triggers switch roles, making it a lot harder for you to manage either one.

All the symptoms of RLS with respect to these psychological conditions have been associated with increased nerve impulses. Of course, it is impossible to determine how exactly the mind can increase the symptoms of this physical condition. Some tests also suggest that an impact on the immune system due mental stress and anxiety could lead to increased symptoms of not just RLS but several other physical conditions as well.

8. Other Triggers

There are several other triggers for RLS. These triggers may not necessarily cause RLS. However, when you already have the condition, these triggers may make the symptoms worse and unbearable. It is a good idea to control or entirely eliminate the following triggers when you have been diagnosed with even possible RLS.

Nicotine

Well, there is a bright side to everything, including RLS. In most cases, RLS is the perfect excuse to stop smoking. Nicotine is basically the addictive substance that is present in tobacco. It can be consumed in many forms including cigarettes and also by chewing tobacco. While there is no research as such to support the fact that nicotine can increase restless leg syndrome, it has been anecdotally stated by many doctors and patients that quitting smoking has been one of the most successful steps towards improving RLS symptoms. It is recommended that you give this a shot, too.

Caffeine

Caffeine is known to be a stimulant that can interfere with our sleep cycle. When caffeine is consumed just before falling asleep or even too close to bed time, it may result in an inability to fall asleep. This can be a very strong trigger for your RLS symptoms. When you are on medication, especially, you must avoid RLS. Research states that caffeine makes it harder for your cells to absorb the medication. That is why; many of the doctors who treat you might recommend that you get off caffeine during your treatment.

Alcohol

While alcohol is usually considered to induce sleep, the effects can be quite contrary with respect to RLS. In case of any sleep disorder, including sleep apnea, it is a common observation that alcohol interferes greatly with the sleep cycle, making it impossible for you to fall asleep. According to Aldo Alvin, the director of the Sleep Disorders Clinic at ULCA, this adverse effect of alcohol has been reported by many individuals with sleep disorders. While there is no solid proof to support this hypothesis, many individuals with RLS have reported that they feel fresh and well rested when they avoid alcohol before going to bed.

Exercise

The relationship between RLS and exercising is still highly debated. Some studies suggest that vigorous exercise just before you go to sleep or close to bed time can make your symptoms worse. Still, other hypotheses say that RLS is a condition that arises due to inactivity. The best conclusion that you may derive from this is that moderate and relaxing exercises can help you stay free from the symptoms. Of course, you must indulge in basic activities like walking or even stretching in order to reduce the symptoms caused by Restless Leg Syndrome.

So, you see, there are so many causal factors of RLS. However, every one of them is still under scrutiny as the exact association with RLS has still not been pointed out for all these symptoms. It is sometimes quite astonishing how little we know about this condition that affects 10% of the general population in the USA alone!

Chapter 8: Treatments for RLS

Initially, you will probably be able to only describe the painful and creepy sensations in your leg. Now, as I've already mentioned, this is one condition that even many health practitioners may not be able to diagnose accurately. If you are suspecting RLS, make sure you tell your doctor that. In many cases, they may simply give you sedatives or medicines to relieve you from the pain. While these medicines may work temporarily, they will do nothing to cure your condition completely. So, even with the slightest doubt, make sure you get diagnosed for RLS.

In case you visit a sleep clinic, they will probably be able to help you with RLS better. Today, most doctors follow the International Restless Leg Syndrome Rating Scale to evaluate the severity of the symptoms. You will be given a questionnaire that will ask you specific questions about your symptoms. Based on the answers that you provide, you will be scored. This test will not only determine the severity of your symptoms but will also act as the first step towards diagnosing the condition.

There are a few questions that are commonly asked in the questionnaire. Here is what you can expect when you go for an evaluation of your RLS symptoms:

• An overall rating of the discomfort that you experience in your legs or in other parts of your body.
• An overall rating of the urge you feel to move around when you experience these symptoms.
• A rating of the relief you experience after you move the body part where you experience the discomfort.
• A rating of the severity of the sleep disturbance that you experience because of RLS.
• Do you feel tired? If yes, how tired do you feel whenever your RLS symptoms show up?

- How would you rate your condition overall?
- Do you feel the symptoms regularly?
- On an average day, how bad can the symptoms get?
- How much does this condition interfere with your ability to carry out your daily activities? Does it cause discrepancies in your family, your school or at your workplace?

The above questions must be rated as mild, moderate, severe, very severe or none at all. Based on the answers you provide, you will be scored and the treatment for your condition will be provided accordingly.

What to Tell your Doctor?

When you suspect that you have RLS, you must be able to explain the symptoms effectively to your doctor. Here are four things that you must keep in your mind when you visit a doctor for the first time:

1. Explain how the symptoms feel: There are different ways of explaining how you feel when you get these symptoms. The most common and easiest to understand explanation is feeling a creeping and crawling sensation in your legs along with tingling in your toes. Be sure to tell your doctor what happens when you move around? Do the symptoms diminish and come back as soon as you stop the movement?

2. How badly is RLS affecting your sleep and your productivity: You must explain when your symptoms get worse. Is it only when you go to bed or do they occur whenever you try to get some rest? You must also tell your doctor if these symptoms keep you up at night. If you are unable to fall asleep or even remain asleep, make sure you bring it to the notice of your doctor. The RLS symptoms must be severe at night but sometimes it feels like the symptoms just don't go away. Mention both to your doctor.

3. Are you taking any medicines currently? You might already be consuming some medicine to relieve yourself of the RLS symptoms. It is also possible that you are taking some other pain killer that may not be related to RLS. You must be clear about this with your doctor to make sure that there is no interference with the medicines that he may prescribe. If any medicines that you consumed in the past made your symptoms worse, tell your doctor about it. You may also request for medicines that do not have as many side effects as the medicines you are already consuming.

Your doctor may also ask your questions about your work and your emotional state. Make sure you answer all these questions accurately so that a proper diagnosis can be done to provide the right kind of treatment to help you overcome RLS symptoms.

1. Treatment Options

The primary goal of any RLS treatment is to reduce the symptoms experienced by the person. This is done to ensure that he or she can get better sleep. The severity of RLS symptoms is related to sleep apnea caused by Restless Leg Syndrome. The stress caused due to this condition is often responsible for the increase in the symptoms. There are two types of therapies that are recommended for RLS:

Non pharmacological Therapy: As the name suggests, these treatment options do not have any type of medicine. The primary goal of these treatments is to ensure that the symptoms are reduced. With these treatment options, there is very little clinical evidence to support them. The systematic trials are available for them are also very few. These methods usually consist of simple lifestyle changes that one needs to make in order to avoid the triggers for these symptoms.

Pharmacological Therapy: There are several medicines that have been used to reduce RLS symptoms. My doctor gave me some tablets to take and that is the main reason why I started my "big investigation" into what else I could to, without taking medication. I simply didn't like the idea of taking medication for the rest of my life for my RLS. I did take some medication, one of them being Amitriptyline 10mg but that didn't work. The doctor said I should try to up the doses, so go to 20mg instead of 10mg. Now I realise, once I go to 30mg, and that doesn't work, the doctor will suggest to go to 40mg, then 50mg, etc.... As most medication like this can be addictive, I decided to stop using it.

These medicines are usually dopamine receptor agonists that activate the receptors, helping the neurons transmit messages easily. The production of dopamine and the consequent effect on the iron level in the body is also managed with these medicines. Several dietary supplements may also be used as part of treatment in order to provide the nutrients necessary to prevent RLS symptoms.

Both these treatment options have been discussed in complete detail in the next section of this book.

Treating RLS with Medicines

The clinical evidence available for the treatment of RLS is very little. There are also very few studies that have been conducted to evaluate the effect of certain medicines on this condition. Even the ones that have been conducted are limited to about 20 patients in the study group, making it hard to quantify these studies and estimate their trend in a general population. There are several reasons why these studies are so small. First, the lack of awareness leads to some bias as the symptoms are noticed only by those with severe RLS. So, they are the only ones who actually participate in these tests. Second, if you want to conduct a polysomnographic test, the patients must sleep in the lab for at least one night. This is very expensive and requires the time of the technicians involved. The absence of resources and the reluctance on the part of the individuals participating in the test, has led to a lack of clinical evaluation.

For a very long time, the tests that were conducted used to compare the study group to a baseline data available. This made it difficult to offer any new findings. In other tests, the patients were given higher doses of a particular medicine till the symptoms were completely gone. This led to severe adverse effects later on, rendering the medicine useless as a form of treatment.

The methods that are used to verify the subjects differ largely from one test to another. Therefore, it is also difficult to compare two studies as the basics itself are so different. Some tests use the rating scales to evaluate the results obtained. Others are based on the limb activity and the awakening of the person at night. There was no method of self-assessment that could be used in these tests until the year 2003!

There were also not many ways to accurately understand the possible adverse effects of the potential therapeutic agents. The studies conducted are so small in size that it becomes extremely difficult to measure any adverse effects at all. Usually, it is accepted that the adverse effects of a particular drug are the same irrespective of the condition it is used to treat. However, in case of RLS exclusive adverse effects have been observed, making it necessary to conduct more studies. In many studies, there is no mention of the adverse effects at all. This makes the unavailability of information more.

One of the most common methods of patient evaluation for RLS is to study their ferritin concentration. Along with this, even the haemoglobin level, the RBS count etc. are determined. This is because the symptoms of RLS are usually experienced by individuals who have low ferritin levels in their body. With iron supplementation, the symptoms have been considerably reduced. However, it was also noted that for patients without frank iron deficiency, these medicines did not show any effects. Currently, the information available on the treatment procedures is very limited. Here are some common medicines that your doctor may recommend to help relieve you of these symptoms.

Iron Supplements

There is no study with a placebo control that can evaluate the effects of oral iron supplements in individuals with RLS. There are studies which compare the intake of Intravenous doses of iron dextran with a placebo. These tests were conducted on individuals with End Stage Renal Failure. These patients were observed for about an hour after administering these medicines. When these tests were conducted over a week, it was revealed that the RLS symptoms actually reduced considerably with these medicines. During the second week, the symptoms peaked and then they declined drastically thereafter. Iron replacement as a secondary RLS treatment has no consensus as yet. In many clinics, 200 mg of elementary iron supplements are given to individuals with anaemia. The medicines are divided into several doses as per the capability of the patient. There are some side effects like:

- Dark Faeces
- Nausea
- Diarrhoea
- Vomiting

This makes oral medication complicated. There may be several other side effects that could stay long term if the medication is consumed for long periods of time. Nevertheless, iron supplementation is one of the first recommended pharmacological treatments available for RLS. When consumed in the standard doses, these medicines may not have as many adverse effects.

Dopaminergic Agents

These are the most preferred medications provided for individuals with RLS. Here are some types of Dopaminergic agents that may be used to treat RLS:

Levodopa

This is one of the most extensively studied oral medicines for Restless Leg Syndrome. It contains a substance known as dopa decarboxylase inhibitor. This substance prevents the conversion of this medication into dopamine. It also crosses the blood brain barrier to treat the condition effectively.

For this medication, there are several tests available to confirm its reaction on RLS symptoms. Three of these tests are placebo controlled as well. In one of the studies, a test group of 28 patients with idiopathic RLS were evaluated for a period of four weeks. Their response to these medications was assessed on the basis of a sleep diary, an actigraphy and a polysomnography. Towards the second week, it was observed that the periodic limb movements of these individuals reduced significantly. They also noted that their sleep quality and the duration of their sleep increased over time. There was an overall improvement in the quality of life of these patients who reported that they were no longer feeling negative feelings and the urge to complain.

In another study, 35 patients were given a version of levodopa called benserazide levodopa. The study was evaluated with a control placebo group. For a period of four weeks, the periodic limb movements were studied. Based on the response, the dose was also adjusted. It was noted that there was a significant decline in the number of periodic limb movements per hour. This improvement was seen as early as on the first day of administering the drug, providing some hope for individuals with RLS.

It is also important to understand who is eligible for benserazide levodopa. This was studied by von Scheele and Kempi. They noted that out of 30 patients in a study group, 9 of them noticed a decline in the symptoms. For 2 patients, the effect was lost after using the medication for about one month. For others, the number of awakenings in the night reduced quite drastically and allowed better sleep duration as well.

Dopamine agonists

These are the most widely recommended medicines for individuals with RLS. According to the studies available, there are three agents that have provided the best results among patients with RLS. These three agents are:

- Ropinirole: This was the first RLS medicine that was approved by the Food and Drug Administration. There were four tests that provided significant data about the use of this drug in controlling the symptoms of RLS. Most of these tests used oral ropinirole as the subject of the study. The results were evaluated on the basis of the IRLS rating scale, the Global Impression Improvement scale and the reports of the patients. The challenge of these tests was to generate a change in the IRLS rating of these patients.

It was also noted that the sleep pattern improved in most of these patients significantly. There were some adverse effects that were noted including nausea and headache.

- Pergolide: Oral doses of this medicine have shown significant results in patients with RLS. This is one of the most successful medicines used in controlling RLS. Although there are few clinical trials with large groups to evaluate this medication, the results obtained have been significant enough to administer this as an effective medication.

One of the most important tests conducted involved 100 patients who were compared to a placebo control group for a period of 6 weeks. It was noted that 68 patients responded positively to pergolide. The study was then extended for one year and the subjects were given an opportunity to participate in this study. The observation was that the effect of the drug was seen even after a period of one year, making it a long term treatment option.

- Pramipexole: There are fewer studies available to support the benefits of pramipexole. It was noted that periodic limb movements reduced by 98% when this medicine was administered. For the others the medicine was partially effective. Although this cannot be used as enough elucidation for the effects of this medicine, it was noted that RLS symptoms were controlled for up to 2 years with this dopamine agonist.

The primary role of dopamine agonists is to interact with the dopamine receptors in our brain. Usually RLS symptoms manifest when the number of receptors is reduced or when these receptors are damaged. These medicines are great to stimulate the receptors to enable proper binding of the dopamine that is produced. So, the body does not respond as if there is a dopamine deficiency and the production of this neurotransmitter is restored to its normal level.

Anticonvulsants

There are several anticonvulsants that have been used to treat RLS successfully. They have been tested using placebo controlled clinical trials. The commonly recommended anticonvulsants for RLS are valporic acid, carbamazepine and gabapentin. These medicines control the impulse transmissions in our spinal cord. Additionally, they also play an important role in dopamine and serotonin production. These two neurotransmitters have an effect on the RLS symptoms. In case of painful symptoms, gabapentin has been prescribed the most as it helps control the pain. There are some adverse effects of anticonvulsants including nausea and sleepiness.

Opioids

While opioids are used very often to feel relief from the symptoms of RLS, there is no substantial proof to support the use of these agents. There are only two opioids, namely propoxyphene and oxycodone that have some research to back them. Even these studies have been conducted only on smaller groups and do not have as much data about them. Tramadol is another opioid that has been used to treat RLS. This medicine has been prescribed based on the testimonials presented by individuals who have taken this medicine before.

Benzodiazepines

Benzodiazepines have been used extensively in the past as a treatment for RLS. Of all the benzodiazepines available, the one that has been studied the most is Clonazepam. There are three small studies that have been used to evaluate the effects of this medicine. The largest test conducted consisted of 13 RLS patients. They were given one dose of clonazepam and were compared with a placebo group. It was noted that the number of awakenings reduced significantly and the sleep quality of these individuals improved with time, as well.

Medication I have been prescribed:

- Gabapentin 300mg Capsules - take 2 at night.

- Pramipexole Dihydrochloride - 125mg - take 1 at night.

Precautions During RLS Treatment

As you have seen for most of the medicines that have been administered for RLS, there are no exact clinical scores or results to evaluate the effects. In addition to that, the adverse effects are not well known as the study groups are seldom over 100 individuals. For this reason, you must be careful about a couple of activities when you are undergoing treatment for RLS as your body may react quite differently.

Here is one important tip for anyone who is trying RLS medicines. *Never believe that the medicine will have the same effect on you as it did on someone else.* The reason is that you do not know the exact causal factor for you and you are not even sure of the adverse effects that you may have as a result of a certain medicine.

Never drive after taking your RLS medication: There are chances that you will notice how a certain medicine affects you only after taking it for at least for one month. Until you are entirely sure of the side effects of a certain medicine, you must never drive. There are chances that you will feel dizzy or sleepy as a result of these medicines. You can also have impaired reflexes and temporary loss of coordination when you take these medicines. So, you must always ask your healthcare provider when it would be appropriate for you to continue with these activities.

Do not operate heavy machines: All the reasons mentioned above are valid enough to prevent you from operating any heavy machines. In case your job involves using machines, it would be best for you to take a couple of days off or request for some time off the machines. If you can get a letter from your doctor, this should be possible. You will need an approval from your doctor before you start using any machinery to avoid injuries or accidents due to the adverse effects of your medicines.

Do not take other medicines that make you sleepy: The role of most RLS medicines is to make sure that you are able to fall asleep better. So, naturally they will make you feel sleepy and drowsy. So, unless it is recommended by your doctor, do not consume any other medicine that may increase your sleepiness or drowsiness. This will have a prolonged effect and can also lead to lack of coordination and slow thinking eventually. Although these effects are not permanent, they may interfere with your performance and can affect your relationships at home, at school or even at work.

Never ignore suicidal thoughts: I have seen that many individuals who consume RLS medications have suicidal thoughts after consuming a particular drug for a long period of time. You must pay close attention to any change in your mood or in your behaviour. Even with the slightest change in your thoughts, contact your healthcare provider immediately.

Here are some common observations among people who experience a change in their thoughts when they take RLS medicines:
- They have constant thoughts of committing suicide. They may even attempt to commit suicide.
- Feelings of depression and anxiety become worse with the consumption of medicines.
- They may feel overly aggravated or irritated.
- Sleep becomes even harder. They may experience worse insomnia.
- They tend to be more violent. It is possible that they are extremely impulsive in all their actions.
- They tend to talk too much or even show bouts of mania. The levels of activity may increase abnormally

If you notice these changes or anything similar, make sure you talk to your doctor.

Do not stop any medication on your own: When you notice suicidal thoughts or any other side effects due to your medication, it is not the best idea to stop this medicine on your own accord. Sometimes, there may be other underlying factors that are actually responsible for your mood swings. In fact, it is possible that your side effects increase drastically when you stop taking these medicines. So, make sure you talk you your doctor first.

Pay attention to allergic reactions: There may be some allergic reactions such as blisters or rashes on your skin. Make a note of these reactions and talk to your doctor without fail. Even the slightest allergy could mean that there could be serious effects on your liver or your kidneys. These are the symptoms that you must look out for:
- Hives
- Swelling of the lips

- Yellowing of the eyes
- Sudden fatigue
- Severe pain in your muscles
- Frequent infections
- Swollen glands that are persistent
- Rashes

You must call your doctor immediately when you notice these symptoms. They could be signs of a serious reaction that could even be fatal. In fact, before any medication is administered to you, a thorough check up to test for allergies should be done first. If you notice these symptoms even after you have been tested for allergies, you need to bring it to the notice of your healthcare provider.

Never replace medicines on your own: Even though two medicines have the same function, they may have extremely different effects on the body as their mechanism of working on the RLS symptoms could be different. So even if you are replacing one dopamine agonist with another, consult your doctor first. Though they are medicines in the same category, the receptors that they stimulate are entirely different. Of course, if you are replacing an anticonvulsant with an opioid, it goes without saying that you must not do this on your own. Since these medicines affect your nervous system, remember to never self-prescribe medicines.

Tell your doctor about all the medicines you are consuming: It is not necessary that these medicines are related to RLS. No matter what medication you are taking, tell your healthcare practitioner. In case you have diabetes or high blood pressure, you may be taking prescription medicines on a regular basis. For women, the relaxants taken during their menstrual cycle should also be reported. Medicines may not only interfere with the effect produced by a certain medicine but may also amplify the side effects that are caused by a certain medicine.

Avoid alcohol when you are on RLS medicines: Alcohol by itself has the ability to increase the symptoms of RLS. So, it may interfere with the effect produced by a certain medicine. There are also chances that any side effect is aggravated when you consume medications along with alcohol. You can ask your healthcare practitioner if small amount of alcohol are permitted.

When you are undergoing treatment for RLS, make sure you bring the following to the notice of your doctor:
- Kidney problems if any. Tell your doctor if you are on hemodialysis.
- Any depression, anxiety, suicidal thoughts, behavioural issues or mood swings that you may have had in the past
- Seizures, if you have experienced any or currently have
- Any history of drug abuse
- Your plans of becoming pregnant or if you are currently expecting a baby. There are some medicines that will be safe to consume even when you are pregnant. Even if you are breastfeeding, you must bring it to the notice of your doctor so that appropriate medicines can be given to you.

There are other side effects such as headaches, nausea, vomiting etc. that may be noticed with your RLS medications. You must be alert about all these effects and bring them to the notice of your doctor for better treatment.

Keep a Sleep Diary

This can be an important aid during your RLS treatment. A sleep diary can work really well and can help you keeping track of the effect that a certain medicine has on you. There are various types of diaries that you can maintain. You will also find mobile applications that will help you track your sleep. A simple log works best to determine the quality of your sleep and also the details of your RLS symptoms. The sleep diary should be filled out when you wake up and just before you go to bed. You can have a standard set of topics that you will address each time to maintain a consistency in all your logs. This is what you can do:

When you wake up:

There are some things you can list when you wake up:

- The time you woke up
- The time you got out of bed
- The time your RLS symptoms began
- The severity of the symptoms: rate them between 1 to 5, 1 being mild and 5 being severe
- The time you fell asleep again
- The number of awakenings
- The total number of hours you've slept

Before you go to bed:

- Daytime RLS symptoms, if any
- The time at which you experienced these symptoms
- How severe were the symptoms, again on a scale of 1 to 5
- The biggest stress for the day
- If you've consumed any alcohol, caffeine, prescription drugs or any other substance.
- How many times you've consumed these substances
- No. of hours you've exercised
- Any specific comments about the day

At the end of every week you review these logs and make a list of questions for your doctor. This makes your check-ups more effective. Also, your doctor can assess if the medication that he is providing is having the desired effects. If there are any new developments after a certain medicine is prescribed, it allows your doctor to make changes in your prescription accordingly.

I know that when you have RLS, the last thing you want is to have a stressful diary to fill out. It can mess up any chances of getting a few hours of sleep. So, I recommend that you maintain a diary that you can fill up in just a few words. It should be simple, to the point and extremely easy to fill. In some clinics, you will be able to get booklets that you can fill out easily. You also have printable RLS logs that are available online. All these logs are in a tabular form, making it extremely easy for you to fill up.

2. Home Remedies for RLS

WARNING RE OVER THE COUNTER MEDICATION: There are several over the counter drugs like Acetaminophen (Tylenol) or other NSAIDs (Non-steroidal Anti-Inflammatory Drugs) e.g. Ibuprofen, Motrin, Advil and Naproxen medications e.g. Aleve, Anaprox). You must be careful about side effects that can be caused by these medicines. They can cause stomach problems e.g. bleeding and ulcer and they can also cause heart problems. Make sure you consult your doctor before taking any over the counter medication.

If you are worried about the possible side effects of the medicines used to treat RLS, you can try alternative therapies. Some of them have been tried and tested by doctors as well. However, most of the remedies listed in this book have been recommended by people who have tried them and seen results. A few of them have helped me get rid of the RLS symptoms and fall asleep peacefully. The best thing about home remedies is that there are no side effects like the medicines that are commonly used for treatment. Of course, these home remedies can be used along with traditional treatment methods for faster relief from the symptoms.

All the remedies listed in this book are things that people have tried, people that I have spoken too on forums, when I was researching how to ease my symptoms. Some might work for you, others might not. Give them a try! Which treatment works for you will, of course, depend on the cause of your RLS.

I have added "WORKS FOR ME" to the methods that actually DO work for me. These methods don't completely take away my symptoms but some of the remedies stop my symptoms in it's track. This means that I won't have any symptoms for say 10 to 15 minutes (after that the symptoms would start again). During those 10 to 15 precious minutes, I have the time to fall asleep. Once I am asleep, I usually sleep all night. If I do wake up during the night and I lay down for 5 minutes without actually sleeping, my RLS will kick in again..

All aids mentioned in this chapter can be purchased from Amazon. Just search for it.

1) Deep Tissue Massage: WORKS FOR ME. The novel massages like the hot stone therapies are the ones that can be of great discomfort, or at least they are for me. However, a traditional deep tissue massage with relaxing oils can actually help alleviate the symptoms of RLS. You can either massage your legs, especially the calves, with a lotion or oil on your own or you can opt for scheduled deep tissue massages. These massages relax your muscles entirely, leaving your legs feeling eased. Any stress or emotional distress that you may be experiencing is also reduced with deep tissue massage. You can also have deep tissue massage done by a specialist and that works really well, however, that is very expensive.

2) Placing a Bar of Soap Between the Sheets: WORKS FOR ME: eases the symptoms but doesn't eliminate them. This is a method that several RLS patients swear by. This is an age old practice that has been followed to reduce the symptoms of RLS and provide better rest. There is no scientific proof available to prove the use of soap as a remedy. It is believed that the alkaline properties of the soap could be responsible for this. For some, placing a bar of soap at the end of the bed works while for others, just throwing a bar of soap between the sheets works well. The bar of soap should be fresh and should be mildly scented for best results. Ivory Soap and Dove are recommended by most individuals. You can also get specially medicated soaps that can help you get rid of the symptoms faster.

3) Drink Tonic Water: WORKS FOR ME. For those who experience leg cramps as one of the primary symptoms of RLS, drinking tonic water can be of great use. Of course, you get versions of tonic water that are very high in quinine. Quinine is a relaxant that can reduce nocturnal cramps and tingling sensations as well. This was a popular remedy once upon a time. However, with increasing knowledge about the adverse effects of quinine, it was banned as a remedy for RLS. You can use regular tonic water with a slice of lemon to relieve RLS symptoms. This is particularly useful when you experience cramps and pain in your muscles when you try to fall asleep.

4) Glysolid Cream: WORKS FOR ME. This cream is usually used as a remedy for skin problems. It consists of active ingredients that seep into the skin to remove any cracks or blemishes. This cream also works on the RLS symptoms. It is most probably the hydrating qualities of this cream that relaxes the muscles and eases the pain. It is most effective when you experience burning sensations in your legs or even arms. Downside: stains your sheets and tastes horrible, when accidently touching your mouth with your fingers, after having massaged your feet/legs with the cream.

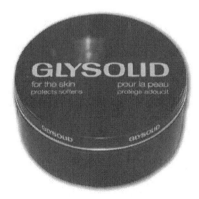

5) Aspirin Tablets: WORKS FOR ME. Besides relieving pain, Aspirin is also known to thin the blood slightly. This improves blood circulation in your legs and throughout the body. As a result, you will see that these "headache tablets" can actually be your saving grace when you are looking for relief from RLS symptoms. I do try and avoid this method as taking aspirin on a regular basis is, I believe, not good for you.

6) Use a Pillow Between Your Legs: WORKS FOR ME. This is a great remedy as you can squeeze the pillow tight and release it when you experience RLS symptoms. This is a relaxation technique that allows better circulation as well. Doesn't take RLS away completely for me, but eases the symptoms.

7) Sand bags in your bed: WORKS FOR ME. When I laid in bed, one evening, I was pushing my foot against my husband's leg, putting some pressure on his leg and to my surprise, I thought: "That actually feels good, it seemed to help my RLS". However, I didn't want to wake up my husband all the time by pushing against his legs! I needed to find something that would fit these 3 purposes:

- An object that wouldn't move when pushed

- A fairly large object, large enough for my feet

- An object that wouldn't disturb my husband on his side of the bed

I came up with the answer: bags of sand! Yes, I do have 2 bags of sand in my bed, wrapped up in a pillow case!

I can say, I am over the moon, as most days, with these three remedies, I do fall asleep and have a good night's sleep:

a) I do stretch exercises first - see remedy number 55.
This is the stretch exercise: Hold on to a door - or something else. Put your feet flat on the floor. Now stand on your tip toes - putting your body weight on your toes - and hold for 3 to 4 seconds and then bring your body down to stand flat on your feet again. Repeat this 20 times: so, on your tip toes, hold for 3 seconds and feet down again - on top toes, hold for 3 seconds and feet down again, etc...You will feel a slight pain in your calf muscles when you do this for the 20th time. When you stand on your toes, make sure you can feel the pressure in your calf muscles. This method works really well for me.

b) Then I massage my feet and calves with Glysolid cream - remedy number 4.

c) Then I push my legs against sand bags - remedy number 7 or put one foot between the two sand bags so the sand bags put a little bit of pressure against my foot.

Hey, sounds silly? This is no joke, this works for me! After years of searching, I've solved my own RLS with bags of sand. By the way, you don't need two bags, one bag might do the job for you but I like pushing both legs against a bag or put one foot against a bag and one foot between the two bags.

Here are some pictures of my sand bags in my bed, so you can see how I position my feet against the bags. I usually put one bag vertically and on bag horizontally in my bed, Reason behind this is that both the bags stay on my side of the bed and don't disturb my husband in his sleep.

On this first picture, I have put my right foot between the two bags of sand and I push the toes of my left foot against the other bag. The pressure on the foot that is between both bags, just feels good.

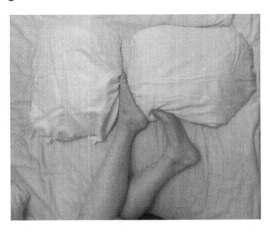

On this picture, I push both feet against the bags:

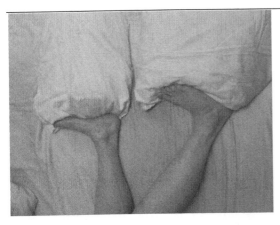

On this last picture, I have moved one bag of sand higher than the other one and push both feet against the bag. So if you like to bend your legs when you go to sleep or not, you can use the bag remedy in both cases.

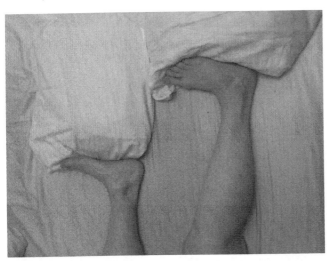

Note: don't push the bag so hard that the bag will actually move. Just push it slightly so you can feel the pressure against your foot.

Now don't ask me to explain medically how it works as I cannot explain it. It just works. I might mention it to my doctor one day and ask him for an explanation.

When I sometimes wake up during the night, with RLS, I repeat these 3 methods again (a,b,c) and it usually works and I fall asleep again almost immediately.

Where to buy these bags of sand? Your local garden centre, you can use a bag of compost or sand. My sand bags are 3 kg each. You can also use the bags that are for sale to fill a children's sand pit. Just search for "bag of sand" in Amazon.

Downside: the bags of sand might damage your mattress. Because of the weight, your mattress might get a dent in it. It has done so on my mattress. I happily accept this though. I'll accept A LOT to get rid of my RLS.

OK, now that you know bags of sand help me, here are some more remedies that might help you.

8) Move Around: Like you already know, moving around is the best remedy to reduce RLS symptoms. Of course, you may not consider this a treatment option. However, when you feel the symptoms at night, you may walk around the house, rub your calves or even kick your legs out in rapid jerks to help relieve the symptoms. In fact, if your symptoms reduce when you move, it is a diagnostic criterion for RLS. You can try to change the pattern of your movement and observe the amount of comfort or ease that you experience when you do so. For some walking helps while for others, the movement needs to be swift and rapid.

9) Trick Your Legs: You can trick your legs to believe that they are still not completely rested. You can do this by wearing your slippers or shoes right until you actually fall asleep. Do not watch television and go to sleep immediately. Instead stretch a little and do some simple exercises just before you go to bed. That way your legs will be under the impression that you are still not rested fully. That way, the symptoms will not aggravate.

10) Walk around before bedtime: Don't go to bed straight away after you've watched a movie on TV - laying down whilst doing so. Instead, walk around for 5 to 10 minutes or do some stretch exercises. Then go to bed.

11) Saliva Works: There is no evidence to suggest how this works but this is a simple and effective method to heal the tingling sensations. Just line a finger with some saliva and rub it on the back of your knee. Rub this up and down for best results. It is possible that the pain relieving property of Saliva helps heal the RLS symptoms as well.

12) Rubbing Magnesium Oil or Lotion on Your Feet: Magnesium deficiency is one of the most important factors when it comes to RLS. It is not necessary to consume magnesium in your diet alone. You can also relieve the symptoms of RLS by rubbing magnesium oil or magnesium lotion on your legs. Both are easily available in any pharmacy or even in your local super market. In some pharmacies, you also get a magnesium spray which is easier to use and a lot more effective in relieving your symptoms. The magnesium required for your body is absorbed through the skin and then utilised.

13) Taking a Nice Hot Shower Before Sleeping: Whether you have a sleeping disorder or not, a nice hot shower is always useful in promoting better sleep. When you have restless leg syndrome, you can fall asleep comfortably when you take a shower. Try to direct the water to your calves or your problem areas. The muscles are relaxed, relieving you of the creepy sensations and the pain that is common when you have RLS. Hot water also helps improve blood circulation, making the symptoms milder. Most often, the stiffness in the muscles is caused due to lack of proper circulation.

14) Rubbing Vitamin E oil on the Legs: Vitamin E is responsible for proper blood circulation in our body. In addition to this, there are several other functions like protecting the tissues in the brain, allowing them to transmit signals better. Of course, when you are using Vitamin E as a home remedy, the reason you will feel relief immediately is because circulation is improved.

Thus, the hardening of the muscle also reduces relieving sensations like the creepy crawly feeling in the legs and the excruciating pain. The increased blood circulation may also provide relief from the periodic limb movements that occur when we have fallen asleep.

15) Vitamin B Supplementation: Vitamin B plays an extremely important role in regulating the iron that is present in the body. So if you have an iron deficiency, using Vitamin B supplements can help relieve the symptoms to a large extent. In addition to that, these supplements also induce the production of certain neurotransmitters that are responsible for enabling proper motor function in the body. Vitamin B deficiency often goes unnoticed. It is a good idea to take tablets containing Vitamin B12 on a regular basis. If you are a vegetarian, especially, your chances of having a Vitamin B deficiency are much higher as meats form the best source of natural Vitamin B12.

16) Tie a Bar of Soap on the Calf: This method has dual purposes. To begin with, the soap acts, as mentioned above. Also, tying your calf gently when you go to sleep also keeps your muscles held as you sleep. This reduces the common sensations that you experience such as creepy feeling or even excruciating pain. In fact, this also allows you to stay in contact with the bar of soap all night. When you just keep the soap at the end of the bed, it may fall off. For many people I know, not having that bar of soap nearby can be distressing.

17) Consider Replacing Your Mattress: There could be a big chance that it is your mattress that is aggravating your symptoms. If you have a very soft mattress, you tend to sink into it while you sleep. This restricts your movement when you are sleeping, making your symptoms worse. Instead, you can use an in spring mattress that allows you to stay on the surface, permitting you to move better. Remember, one of the most common triggers for RLS is being completely at rest. IF your mattress is somewhat "trapping" you, it is a good idea to swap it with a more solid one.

18) Cleanse Your Feet: This method is also called an energising cleanse. The idea is simple, make a mixture of baking soda in a tub of warm water and wash the feet and the areas that are affected by the RLS symptoms. This process relaxes your muscles completely. In addition to that, even your blood circulation improves drastically. For some of my friends, a complete cleansing ritual is important. This means that they also need to clean up the space that they will be sleeping in to feel the effect of this method. You can try whatever works for you!

19) Soak Your Feet in Epsom salts: Epsom salts have always been known for their ability to relax the muscles. For any soreness in your feet or your legs, you can soak your feet in a tub of warm water containing Epsom salts. Of course, these salts are also useful in improving the blood circulation in your legs. In addition to this Epsom salts also contain magnesium that is extremely essential for those who are suffering from symptoms of RLS. However, you must never over use Epsom salts as the results are quite adverse leading to skin problems and other such issues. So, use this only when the symptoms are severe.

20) Apply Aloe Vera Gel: Aloe Vera has extremely relaxing properties that can soothe your muscles. This relieves you of cramping and pain, thus reducing the symptoms of RLS. For some, even the mild smell of aloe Vera acts as a relaxant and helps them sleep better.

21) Baking Soda: When your legs are sore or have cramps, there is a heavy accumulation of lactic acid in that region. Using an antacid like baking soda can relieve the pain almost instantly. You can dissolve a teaspoon of baking soda in half a glass of water and drink it. You can even make a more concentrated solution and rub it on the affected area for immediate results.

22) Splash Cold Water on the Calves: For many of my friends, cold water is the only answer to their symptoms. This works only when the sensations have already started in the legs. It is a common assumption that this method works because the muscles are shocked with the cold water. They are crunched for a moment because of the cold water and relieved immediately. That way the muscles relax, leading to complete relief from the symptoms. You can also try a cold ice pack. It has the same effect as cold water but the effect is more and also localised.

23) Wet Socks for Burning Feet Sensations: One of the worst sensations associated with RLS is known as hot feet. This is when you experience unpleasant burning sensations in the feet all night long. A very simple remedy was recommended by one of the members of an online forum. He explains how wearing wet socks can relieve these symptoms completely. If you don't feel comfortable despite this, another option is to direct a fan towards your feet when the socks are on. Of course, this is not necessary during the colder months or during monsoons. However, if your burning sensations are severe, you can try this to see the difference.

24) Hot and Cold Treatment: Hot and cold treatment is a way of shocking your muscles. You can apply a heat pack and alternate it immediately with an ice pack. This relieves contracted muscles and you will notice that the spasms and the contractions in your legs will disappear. You can even try the same on any part of your body that is affected by the RLS symptoms. You may even try alternating between a hot and a cold shower. You can alternate them every 20 to 30 seconds and keep the shower about 5 minutes long. This can even relax your entire nervous system instantly.

25) Lidoderm Pain Patches: These patches are usually recommended for viral damage caused to the nerves. It is known for relieving the painful symptoms caused by this condition which is known as postherpetic neuraglia. This patch comes with an adhesive and can be applied on the affected region before sleeping or even during the day to find relief from the symptoms.

26) Cold Pack: You can apply an ice pack on your legs when you are about to go to bed. There are other ways to decrease the temperature. You can place your socks in the freezer all day and wear them when you go to sleep. You can even wrap ice in a sock and gently rub it over your legs. This improves blood circulation and thus relieves you from the tingling sensations that are common with RLS.

27) Evening Primrose Tablets: Primrose tablets contain natural extracts that are known to ease skin problems. This tablet is also recommended for rheumatoid arthritis. It is known to reduce nerve damage when consumed for 6 to 8 months consistently. Primrose tablet can also ease conditions that lead to RLS including liver damage and peripheral neuropathy. So, this is a popular home remedy among RLS patients.

28) Heel Cups: You can wear heel cups in your shoes to ease RLS symptoms. With heel cups, the strain on your heels and ankle is reduced considerably. They also align your bones giving you proper posture all day. This can help relieve the RLS symptoms as the legs are more relaxed and stress free all day.

29) Use Aerowalkers: When you are resting or just sitting in one position for long hours, using an aerowalker can be of great use. The primary function of aerowalkers is to improve circulation in your legs. They work with a simple reflex action that takes place without your attention. So, while you are reading a book or watching TV, these aerowalkers help increase circulatory activity in your feet, reducing the RLS symptoms.

30) Increase Omega 3 intake: Omega 3 is known to reduce any stiffness or tenderness in your joints. Studies reveal that Omega 3 has the ability to prevent inflammation and destruction of cells in the body. They also inhibit cytokines that are responsible for inflammation. This helps reduce the RLS symptoms to a large extent. Eating fish or taking fish oil supplements can help. If you are vegan or vegetarian, you can eat 5 to 6 walnuts with water every morning.

31) Place your Feet Higher Than the Head: This is a simple thing you can do when you go to bed. Just place your feet on a pile of pillows or on a foam cushion. This ensures better circulation of blood and also keeps your feet supported when you are sleeping, reducing RLS symptoms.

32) Use Better Footwear: Wearing high heels or ill fitted shoes can cause damage to your muscles and also the nerve endings in your feet. Make sure your shoes have enough support and also good shock absorption in order to reduce the strain on your legs. Good shoes also ensure better posture, reducing the intensity of RLS symptoms.

33) Massaging the Leg with Salt and Coconut Oil: Coconut oil has several benefits. One of these is the cooling effect that it has on the muscles when it is used for a massage on a regular basis. Coconut oil is recommended if you have burning sensations in your legs. When you add salt to this massage mixture, you improve the benefits. The salts act as exfoliates; allowing your skin to breathe easily and stay relaxed. A combination of coconut oil and salts can also improve blood circulation in your legs, reducing the cramps, painful sensations and also the creepy sensations that you experience. This is also a very easy home remedy and is recommended by Ayurveda experts

34) Use Muscle Rubs: There are several muscle rubs like Bengay, Tylenol, etc.. that you can use to ease the symptoms of RLS. These muscle rubs are great to relieve the muscles of the strain caused by the RLS symptoms. Another benefit of these rubs is that they help reduce the symptoms of RLS as they increase the blood circulation to the muscles in the region that they are used in. Muscle rubs are easily available and need to be massaged into the problem areas before sleeping every night. Tyenol pm is also recommended by many patients who are suffering from Restless Leg Syndrome.

35) Using Magnetic Insoles: Research shows that magnetic field can improve circulation of blood in your legs. Using magnetic insoles are great when you experience intense RLS symptoms. The only thing you need to remember is that these insoles need some maintenance. Since the minerals in your sweat can damage the insoles, you may have to wash them with warm water and soap every day and dry completely before using. You can place these insoles in your socks every night as a remedy for RLS symptoms.

36) Reduce Sweets and Sugars: You must cut out sweets and sugars after 4pm. It is seen that RLS symptoms and cramping can aggravate as a result of sugar in your blood stream when you are going to bed.

37) Take a break: When you are working, make sure you take small breaks of at least 5 mins of and on. This is necessary especially when you have a secretary job or a job that requires you to stand for several hours. This will keep your legs moving and exercised to reduce RLS symptoms.

38) Use Fenugreek Seeds: Fenugreek seeds are a great remedy for joint pain and also for kidney problems. Fenugreek also allows you to keep your weight in check. You can soak a few seeds in water at night and consume the water in the morning. You can also soak fenugreek seeds in mustard oil and apply it on the affected area for relief from RLS symptoms.

39) Walk Around With Flip Flops Before Sleeping: When you wear flip flops, there are several minute actions that your muscles perform in order to keep the flip flops in place. So walking around with them will stimulate the muscles in your feet. This helps reduce the RLS symptoms.

40) Stay Hydrated: Drink lots of water all day. Instead if drinking water at once, take small sips all day. Water is a great antioxidant. It reduces free radicals in your body that cause RLS symptoms. When you keep yourself hydrated all day, the muscles even the absorption of essential minerals and nutrients improve. Water soluble minerals like Vitamin B require a good supply of water in order to be used effectively by the body.

41) Try Exercises That Stimulate the Mind: One of the most common causes of RLS is the inactivity of the neurons. Whether

111

it is because the receptors of the neurotransmitters that experience problems or whether it is the physical condition of the neuron itself, any damage to the neuron can cause RLS symptoms. One of the simplest ways to relieve yourself of these symptoms is to makes sure that you keep your mind stimulated at all times. You may try simple exercise like puzzles, Sudoku and crosswords that keep you stimulated mentally. You can also indulge in word games like scrabble as they require you to apply your mind to play. Make it a habit to spend a couple of hours stimulating your mind. Several other activities like reading can also help. In addition to relieving RLS symptoms, these activities also help you reduce stress.

42) Sip Chamomile Tea Before Sleeping: Chamomile tea is a very relaxing drink that you may consume before going to bed. It is a very good antioxidant that provides other benefits for your health as well. Chamomile tea is herbal and is therefore extremely safe to use. The antioxidising properties of chamomile are also useful in preventing oxidative damage to your RBCs. This reduces any chances of an iron deficiency in your body. Additionally, Chamomile is also known to induce sleep. Thus, the quality of your sleep improves along with the number of hours you are able to sleep peacefully.

43) Add Fennel To Your Diet: This is another Ayurveda remedy that has been brought to my notice through testimonies presented on RLS blogs online. You can consume fennel in many ways. You may include it in your diet, consume the seeds like tablets or even soak the seeds overnight and drink the water in the morning. Fennel is a cooling agent. So, it is extremely useful when you are experiencing burning sensations in your legs as an RLS symptom. Fennel is also a relaxant. If your weight is an issue for your RLS symptoms, fennel is a great option as it helps you burn fat and reduce the kilos.

44) Valerian Root: If the carefully processed roots of the Valeria plant are available, they are extremely useful in controlling RLS symptoms. Most often valerian root is consumed in the form of a tea. You can also buy tonics or capsules containing extracts of valerian root. This is another herbal remedy. However, there have been several side effects of valerian root because of which doctors advise you to consult a specialise before consuming it. Valerian root is known for its sedative properties. It is one of the most highly recommend herbal remedies for any sleep related issue.

45) Use Kava Roots: This is yet another herbal remedy that is very popular with patients who have RLS. Kava is a natural relaxant. This means that you will be able to experience instant muscle relief when you consume kava supplements. You will also notice that consuming this root's extracts help you fall asleep faster at nights. Another important benefit that kava root has is its impact on your brain. The extracts of this root can also relax the brain and relieve it from anxiety and stress. Special chemicals present in this root have an immediate effect on the nervous system, relaxing it completely.

46) Black Strap Molasses in a Glass of Water: The primary advantage of black strap molasses is that it is rich is iron. This can help reduce several symptoms of RLS. Like you already know, iron is one of the main components used in the treatment of RLS. If you are suffering from iron deficiency, black strap molasses is the best natural remedy available. Just mix one spoon of black strap molasses into a glass of water. Just half an hour before you go to bed, drink this solution. You must do this every day for the best possible results. Another recommendation is that you use apple cider vinegar in this mixture. However, when you are using apple cider vinegar, make sure that you are not allergic to it.

47) Wear Clothes that Provide Compression: You can get a variety of compression clothing for just your calf muscles and also for your full leg. There are some leading brands like 110 per cent compression that have provided maximum relief for individuals with RLS. You can buy these compression garments from any local medical store as well. The generic versions are cheaper and are quite effective, as well. Before you go to bed, pull the compression garment on. You will notice that the propensity of leg cramping is a lot lesser when you have this garment on. Commonly, individuals with RLS will complain of heaviness in their legs. Even this can be avoided with compression garments. There are special compression socks that are available in the market. These socks are also capable of enabling blood flow in your legs, making you less susceptible to common RLS symptoms.

48) Increase Electrolyte Intake: Many times, the primary cause for the cramping of your muscles is severe loss of minerals from your body. These minerals include potassium, calcium, sodium, iron and magnesium. There are about 80 essential minerals in the body that need to be replenished from time to time to prevent RLS symptoms. You can opt for natural electrolytes to serve this purpose. Some of the best options are drinking mineral enriched water, using Himalayan sea salts, eating fruits and vegetables grown in mineral rich soil etc. There are several mineral rich foods like red meats and also spinach that are recommended for you if you have RLS. You can also avail natural effervescent tablets in sports stores. These tablets dissolve in water easily. They do not contain any sugars that are actually triggers for RLS symptoms. You must avoid the electrolyte drinks that you see in commercials as they are packed with sugars and harmful to your overall health.

49) Use Lavender Essential Oils: Lavender oil is among the most commonly used essential oils. It is considered to be exotic and extremely good for health. One definite health benefit of using lavender oils is the relaxing quality of the oil. For this reason, it has also been tried on RLS symptoms **with** great success. The aroma of lavender oil is extremely calming and is known to help you sleep better. In order to use lavender for relief from RLS symptoms, all you need to do is rub a few drops of this oil on your feet before going to bed. Apply some on each foot for maximum results. You can also pour a few drops of lavender oil into a tub with lukewarm water. Soak your feet in this tub for about ten minutes each day before you fall asleep. This can help you sleep better and also control the RLS symptoms.

50) Peppermint for Stress Relief: The menthol content in peppermint is very high. This has a sort of numbing effect on the uncomfortable feelings that you experience every night. This is also great in relieving any pain in your muscles that is caused due to RLS. You can consume peppermint in several forms. You may drink a warm cup of peppermint tea before you go to bed each night. This will help you get better sleep and will also relax the muscles. For those who suffer from severe RLS, it is also a good idea to consume about 4 cups of peppermint tea every day for maximum relief from the symptoms. You can also apply peppermint to the affected area directly. You will be able to get essential peppermint oils in stores. You can rub these oils on your leg and massage it in for about 15 minutes. The stress in the muscles is relieved almost immediately.

51) Rub Camphor Oils: Camphor has several therapeutic properties. It is known to be a great antispasmodic agent. This means that it can relieve inflammation when used regularly. Inflammation, which is also one of the most important triggers of RLS, is reduced, helping you alleviate the symptoms. All you need to do is apply camphor oil on the affected areas before going to sleep. You will notice that the symptoms vanish almost immediately. You can do this every day for the best possible results. You will also get camphor cream in stores that can be used in the same way to relieve RLS symptoms.

52) Try Apple Vinegar Cider: The primary reason why apple vinegar cider works is because is an alkaline food. Thus, it enables better consumptions of the minerals that are necessary for RLS. You can consume of table spoon of edible apple cider vinegar mixed with a glass of lukewarm water. Sip this water slowly for about half an hour before you go to bed. Some of you may not be able to adapt to the bitter taste. Then, you could opt for the tablets. Another option is that you can apply a small amount of Apple Cider Vinegar on your legs each night before sleeping.

53) Apply Vapo rub: Vapo Rub is also a relaxant that provides heat to your muscles as well. For several RLS patients, using vapo rub has helped curb the RLS symptoms and also improve sleep.

54) Other Remedies: Here are some remedies that have been tried by many with successful results. These methods are effective but there is no explanation for how these methods have helped reduce RLS symptoms. Nevertheless, you may try them. Hopefully, one of them will help you:

- Consume Horse Chestnut Tablets
- Consume 1 teaspoon of diatomaceous earth dissolved in water
- Consume Kratom Leaf Supplements
- Eat a few goji berries or consume their juice
- Use an infrared light beam on the affected area for 30 minutes each day
- Munch on pumpkin seeds
- Eat bananas
- Consume cream of wheat cereal
- Drink only mineral water
- Massage almond oil on the affected area
- Drink water with cinnamon and honey
- Avoid deodorants with aluminium
- Sleep on the floor
- Do not keep a digital clock next to your bed
- Drink a mixture of pineapple juice, tonic water and nutmeg
- Rub alcohol on your feet

So you see there are several simple remedies that you may try at home. These methods are safe, simple and successful. If you are looking for more remedies, try to talk to other individuals who have RLS. If they have tried any home remedies, they should be able to give you some tips. However, make sure that you try each remedy for at least one month before switching to the next. Some of them may give you immediate results, while the others may take longer. You must be consistent with your herbal and natural remedies as well, if you are looking for long term results.

3. Best Exercises for RLS Symptoms

There are several leg stretches that you can do to improve the RLS symptoms or to get temporary relief when the symptoms are too severe. The tightness in your muscles or even the upper body lead to several issues including reduced range of motion, extreme discomfort in the limbs and increased RLS symptoms at night. There are some exercises that are known universally to ease RLS symptoms. Practising them consistently can also lead to complete relief from the symptoms. These exercises are simple and may be done anywhere. Doing them two to three times every day is recommended for definite relief.

WARNING: *NEVER do stretches until it really hurts. You can damage your muscles this way.*

55) Stretch the Calves: WORKS FOR ME. The calf muscles are most prone to the discomfort caused by RLS. In order to relieve the muscle spasms and the pain caused in the calf, you may do a simple stretch regularly. All you have to do is stand facing a wall. Have a distance of about the length of your arm from the wall. Place you palm on the wall. Now, step forward with your right leg. Make sure your left leg is fully straight, with the heel on the floor. Once you have assumed this position, bend your right knee towards the wall. Use your palm to apply pressure and get a better stretch. You should feel the calf muscles in your left leg stretching. Make sure you hold this for at least 30 seconds. Then, repeat this with your other leg as well.

56) Exercise calf muscles: WORKS FOR ME. Hold on to a door - or something else. Put your feet flat on the floor. Now stand on your tip toes - putting your body weight on your toes - and hold for 3 to 4 seconds and then bring your body down to stand flat on your feet again. Repeat this 20 times: so, on your tip toes, hold for 3 seconds and feet down again - on top toes, hold for 3 seconds and feet down again, etc...You will feel a slight pain in your calf muscles when you do this for the 20th time. When you stand on your toes, make sure you can feel the pressure in your calf muscles. This method works really well for me.

57) Stretch your Hamstrings: Stretching the hamstrings can be extremely relaxing. You can either stand straight and roll down to touch your toes for a good stretch or try the doorway stretch. For this, lie down near a doorway. Then place your left leg through the door way and lift the right leg up. Rest your heel firmly on the doorway. Now, continue to lift your right leg with the support of the door way till you can. You must make sure that your right leg is fully straight for a good and thorough stretch. You will feel this stretch all the way down from your back to your hamstrings. Hold this position for about 30 seconds. When you are done, repeat this on the other side as well.

58) Stretch your Quads: Your quads or your quadriceps are your thigh muscles. Stretching them is quite easy. Find a wall and stand with your back against this wall. Now fold one leg in so that the heel touches your buttock. Keep the shoulders pressed against the wall. This will give you a thorough stretch in your quadriceps. Hold this position for about 30 seconds ensuring that your shoulders are touching the wall at all times. When you are through with one leg, make sure you stretch the other one completely too.

When you begin to experience the symptoms of RLS, there are some exercises that will help you get almost immediate relief from the pain and the tingling sensations.

59) Pump the ankles: This is a great exercise to help better blood flow in your legs. You can do this exercise even when you are lying down or just sitting on your chair. In order to perform this exercise, extend your leg in front of the body. Now flex the ankles till your toes point towards your upper body. Then point your toe away from the body. You can repeat this about 20 times. This is an extremely easy exercise to follow. Even when you wake up in the middle of the night due to your RLS symptoms, you can just do these exercises and fall asleep immediately.

60) Walking: This is the next step when the ankle pumps do not work. If your RLS symptoms are extremely painful or severe, walking might provide relief immediately. This will also help you fall asleep quite easily. You see, walking is an exercise that will definitely boost the blood supply to your legs. It is more effective than ankle pumps as the relief to the muscles is a lot more. The blood flow also is more with walking In addition to this, walking is a rhythmic exercise that is extremely relaxing. So, you should be able to fall asleep immediately.

61) Stretch your toes: Lie down and with your legs straight, pull your toes towards you and after that, stretch your toes away from you. Repeat 10 times.

62) Lift your feet: Stand still. Lift up one foot, heel first, followed by ball of your foot and then toes. When on your toes, stretch your foot so you can feel it in your calf muscles hold the foot for 10 seconds and put the foot back to a normal position. Repeat this 10 times with each foot. You can do this exercise even standing in a queue somewhere. This is easy to do but very effective.

63) Legs in the air: Lay on your left side and lift up your right leg in the air, keep it there for 10 seconds and let your leg down again. Repeat 10 times. Do the same laying on your right side and lift up your left leg.

64) Jump: Stand on the floor, feet apart and jump up 10 times. Whilst jumping, it is important to raise your heel first, then your front ball of your foot, and last the toes.

65) Bicycle: Do bicycle exercises in the air with your legs, when lying in bed or on any flat surface.

66) Progressive Relaxation of the Muscles: According to the Best Health magazine, practising progressive relaxation of the muscles just before going to bed can help you. Start by breathing deeply. Then clench or tighten the muscles in your feet. Hold this for a few seconds and relax the muscles completely. Repeat this with your calf muscles. Now work your way up till your head, tensing and relaxing one part at a time. This will help you fall asleep faster as your entire body is relaxed. This also helps when you are stressed or unable to sleep.

When you practice any of these exercises, make sure you do not overdo anything. Stretch only till a point you can. When you feel pain stop immediately. You can also try water exercises like water aerobics and regular swimming for relief from these symptoms.

4. Aids to Relieve RLS

There are several aids that you can use to help reduce the symptoms of RLS.

In order to get a better stretch, you could use a couple of tools. These tools act as assistants and help you safely improve your stretch. Listed below are three simple devices that you can bring home and get a through stretch to improve your RLS symptoms:

67) 3 Bar Leg Stretcher: WORKS FOR ME. As the name suggests, there are three bars in this tool. Two bars are meant for your legs while the third one acts as a support for your hand. You can hold on to this central handle and inch forward. As you do this the legs also open up. This allows you to get a three way stretch. You not only stretch your legs but your entire back as well. This is a very easy to use machine that you can also store quite easily in your home.

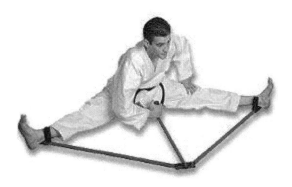

Picture source: www.karatemart.com

68) Resistance Band: This is an elastic band that is mostly used for strength training. However, I have also found it to be extremely useful in stretching the legs and the back. It acts as a great assistant when you want a good and thorough stretch.

69) Heavy Duty Leg Stretcher Machine: This is a heavy machine that is extremely safe to use. You have a good back support in the form of a chair. You can place your legs on the leg rest provided. Then. All you need to do is adjust the handle to increase the distance between the leg rests. As you increase the distance, you have a better stretch. The advantage with this machine is that it is sturdy. You also have ample support and the right posture to ensure that there are no injuries.

70) Foot rockers: These are special shoes with rockers attached to the base. They resemble rocking chairs in their movement. Foot rockers are usually used by athletes to stretch better without any discomfort in the heels and the ankles. They are also great for relieving pain and the tingling sensations experienced when you have RLS symptoms.

71) Heel Cups: You can place these heel cups in your shoes to reduce any shock or stress on your heels. These cups are very useful in aligning you bones and your heel for proper walking and standing posture which is crucial in reducing RLS symptoms.

72) Mobility Lacrosse Ball: When you have strained or tired muscles, you must be feeling sudden relief when you apply pressure on a certain spot. These spots are called fascia. There is a layer of tissue between the muscles that gets knotted and becomes tight when there is no proper movement. Using a lacrosse ball to press into those areas relieves any tension in the affected area. You can work a lacrosse ball down your back and legs for reduced RLS symptoms.

73) Support compression socks and sleeves: Compression socks are known to reduce pain in the legs. These socks can be worn when you experience the RLS symptoms. They provide support to your calf muscles and the nerves running in that region, applying gentle pressure that eases blood flow to relive you of RLS symptoms. You also get special calf sleeves that can provide localised results.

74) Muscle Rollers: There are various types of muscle rollers that you can use to massage your legs, especially the calf muscles.

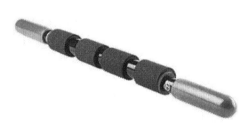

Some of them are:

- Pinpoint Rollers: They have a small rolling ball attached to a handle that you can slide over the affected area. This is used to relieve localised pain.

- Wooden spiked acupressure rollers: These acupressure rollers have wooden spikes   that work on the pressure points on the legs and feet to improve blood circulation and   also   relax   the muscles effectively. These rollers can also be found as acupressure   double foot massager which allow you to relax both the feet at a time.

- Foam rollers: These are soft rollers that can provide relief to a large area each time. You can even relax your muscles before stretching for better results.

- Magnetic handy rollers: These rollers come with magnetic and spiked surfaces with a handle. They also have several types of adjustments that you can make including an unevenly surfaced sujock ball that can relieve strained muscles immediately. The   magnetic effect of the roller ensures better blood flow and reduces the symptoms effectively.

75) Circulation Leg Wraps: These are specialized boots that come with airbags that wrap around the whole leg. You can control the inflation, deflation and the duration of these contractions and expansions. Thus, you also expand and contract your blood vessels. This improves blood blow in your calves, feel, hamstrings and thighs and also your back.

76) Gel Lap Pad: These pads are very useful in preventing and reducing day time symptoms. They are available in various shapes and sizes. They are pads that are filled with a shin and heavy gel that you can place on your lap when you need to sit for several hours. They provide a grounded and secure feeling. They are also ideal for long road trips to prevent RLS symptoms and also manage them. You can stay seated for long hours without any discomfort.

77) Medical Leg Rest: A medical leg rest is a specially cushioned leg rest that is recommended for people with knee pain and also fractures. You can elevate your legs as per your level of comfort to improve circulation and to improve your posture when you have to sit for long hours. You can also keep your leg elevated when you are about to fall asleep. That will help the blood circulate better and will also provide ample support to the muscles in your leg to relieve RLS symptoms.

78) Circulation Improver Machine: These machines stimulate the legs through a rocking action and through vibrations improving circulation in the feet. They activate the blood vessels allowing the legs to contract and relax as the blood is circulated. This healthy form of circulation allows oxygenated blood to reach the legs effectively, relaxing the muscles and relieving you of RLS symptoms. This machine actually made my symptoms worse.

79) Triangular Foam Cushion or Leg Raiser: These are special cushions that you can place directly below the knee joint. Because of their ergonomic shape, they provide enough support to your knees and your legs. This eases any discomfort and reduces the sensations that are common with RLS. Since the leg is fully supported you can relax completely and rest your legs well. You can also ask for orthopaedic pillows.

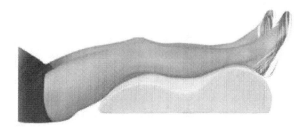

80) Acupressure Mat: Acupressure mats have magnetic points or spikes that can reach out to all the pressure points. You can either stand on the mat for a while or lie down on it for about 20 minutes before you sleep or when you take breaks during your work. The pressure applied relaxes the muscles and improves circulation. This helps alleviate the RLS symptoms or prevents them from appearing at all and also reduces stress. It is known to improve sleep as well.

81) Zero Gravity Lounge Chair: A zero gravity lounge chair is a light, foldable chair that has cushioning from the neck to the foot. The shape of the chair allows you to keep your feet dangling with support at the calf muscles. Therefore, without any stress on your muscles, you can maintain a good posture and experience the benefits of a well-designed chair. This chair is ideal for reading or to watch television as it keeps your back rested at an angle allowing you to relax your entire body. You can sit for several hours without any discomfort.

82) Massagers: There are various types of massagers that you can use before sleeping or during work to reduce RLS symptoms. Some of the most common massagers are:

- Wet Massager: Also known as the motorised food and leg spa bath massager, these massagers allow you to soak your feet in soap water or in Epsom salt while the massager is vibrating and massaging your feet. This allows you to not only enjoy the benefits of a good massage but also experience a great spa like treatment in the comfort of your home.

- Heated massagers: These massagers are great for people who need a good therapeutic foot massage. As the name suggests, these massagers apply heat to your legs to relax strained muscles. They also improve circulation, stimulating your legs. It is a good idea to use this massager just before your fall asleep as the leg feels rested and relaxed.

- Electric Foot Massagers: These massagers use compressions and vibrations that are powered by electricity. You can opt for hand help massagers or the seated massagers. They both work really well and can reduce any pain in your legs. The added benefit is that they guarantee better blood circulation.

- Calf Massagers: These massagers have a cushioned slot where you can rest your entire foot until the calf muscles. Using compression and controlled vibration, these massagers will relive any pain in your calves. They are electrically powered. These are the most effective massagers to reduce any symptom of Restless Leg Syndrome.

83) Have more sex!: RLS and the Libido. If RLS is connected to dopamine, then there must be some connection between our sexual energies and RLS, too. When you experience an orgasm, the dopamine production in your body is on overdrive. That is how you feel the pleasant sensations. Since RLS is so closely linked with dopamine, the next step was to study the effect of sex on RLS. The findings are rather fascinating.

It has been reported that sex, in fact, is one of the most natural remedies for RLS that is available to us. To support this statement, a test was conducted recently. The results of these tests were published in the Sleep Medicine journal. This report was actually the result of a self-discovered cure for RLS. A certain patient had found a very reliable and safe way to relieve himself of RLS symptoms and also fall asleep easily.

The report contains the details of a 41 year old male who suffered from severe RLS. He had been experiencing these symptoms for close to 10 years. He was unable to fall asleep or stay asleep. All the criteria mentioned by the IRLS rating scale had been fulfilled by him. He also had a score of 32 on this scale, confirming that his condition was actually quite severe. He reported that the only time when he was able to get complete relief from the severe symptoms was when he either masturbated or whenever he had sexual intercourse. This is when he was also able to sleep without any night awakening due to the symptoms. As a part of the study, he was given certain RLS medicines to help control the symptoms as well.

He was given pramipexole, a dopamine receptor agonist about 2 hours before he went to bed. The relief was significant. Then, he was deprived of the medication as a part of the study. It was noticed that he simply went back to his sexual behaviour in order to fall asleep and relieve himself of the symptoms that were quite severe. This is one of the only clinical trials to elucidate the role of our libido in Restless Leg Syndrome. There are several anecdotal reports that sexual activity can actually relive a person of the symptoms. On the other hand, there are also reports that suggest that RLS symptoms became worse with sex.

There is no clarity on how the two are related. The only speculations that have been made so far are that the opioids and the dopamine that released in the body during an orgasm could have a significant role to play in relieving even severe symptoms of RLS. There have also been reports of pelvic movements in individuals during the wake and sleep transition. These movements resembled the regular coital behaviour. Of course, these connections do not confirm anything. But it has been reported by several RLS patients that they have had orgasm related effects on their RLS symptoms.

You can buy all the above mentioned aids online. They may also be available in sports stores. When you have an equipment to support you, you are ensured of the right posture. This allows you to push into the stretch further and get the results that you want. The most important benefit of using a machine or a tool is that you can prevent injuries to a large extent.

5. Alternate Therapies for RLS

If you do not believe in conventional medical procedures, there are several alternate therapies for RLS that you may want to try as well. These therapies are safe to try as there are no side effects. Some of the most popular alternate treatment methods for RLS include:

Acupressure

Acupressure is an ancient practice and has been used to relieve symptoms of various conditions experienced by people. There are several pressure points in our body that control the functioning of certain parts of the body. The idea behind acupressure is to locate these pressure points and apply light pressure on them to relieve the tension in the affected area. It is almost like they untie the knots that are formed in the body using these pressure points. The pressure point for RLS syndrome is located at the back of the neck. When you apply pressure on these points, the symptoms are relieved immediately. It is also possible that the symptoms go away completely when you seek acupressure treatment on a regular basis. Acupressure works well on RLS symptoms as it is great to relieve the stress experienced in the body. When these pressure points are addressed, you will feel immediate relief from any anxiety or stress. This leads to relief from the symptoms partially. In addition to that the blood circulation in your body also improves with acupressure. When the respective pressure points are addressed, the blood circulation in the legs also improves instantly. This helps relax the muscles and reduce the pain and the spasms that are experienced commonly. Acupressure is also extremely relaxing, making it a great practice to get better sleep when you suffer from conditions like Restless Leg Syndrome.

Acupuncture

Acupuncture has a significant impact on the neuro hormonal function in our body. This is the perfect combination to relieve RLS symptoms as this is a condition that is affected by the hormonal imbalance in the body as well as the nervous system. This method of treatment relies on finding the right acu points in our body. These points are stimulated by various methods like lifting, pinching and piercing. A modern technique is to stimulate these pressure points is to apply some heat or even weak currents to make the effects show faster. Depending upon the type of acupuncturist you go to the method will differ. In Chinese medication, acupuncture is one of the most popular forms of treatment for RLS. There are certain meridians in the legs that are believed to be obstructed for various reasons. This blockage causes numbness, heaviness and aching sensations in the legs when you have RLS. It is also believed that the internal energy of the person is disturbed causing sleep problems as well. The primary objective of acupuncture is to stimulate the kidneys and the liver. It is believed that this approach improves the flow of blood in the body and also regulates the internal energy. The blockages in the leg meridians are also relieved when acupuncture is used. The selection of the pressure points differs from one individual to another. These pressure pints are chosen based on the flow of energies in the legs. This also promotes better sleep and ensures that your body is in a state of complete rest.

Guided Meditation

Our brain consists of several beautiful images. However, it seems that only the unpleasant ones are voluntarily recalled by us. This causes stress, anxiety and also conditions like Restless Leg Syndrome. On the other hand, if we were to tap into these positive images, we could be able to treat all the unpleasant sensations that we experience with RLS. You can opt for a class or even buy a CD for guided meditation. The idea is to visualise beautiful images as you meditate to enhance your state of mind. You can also imagine pleasant sounds, depending upon the type of guided meditation you have chosen. This method can relieve you of the symptoms of RLS by relaxing your body completely. You will also be able to sleep better when you practice guided meditation. You can do this just before you go to bed to experience the benefits of this wonderful practice.

Clinical Hypnosis

Clinical hypnosis is a great mind and body therapy that can be used to get to the bottom of the cause for your RLS symptoms. It is believed that through hypnosis, one can will himself to prevent the periodic limb movements at night. You can also use the power of your mind to relieve yourself from the painful and uncomfortable sensations caused by RLS. The exact relationship between RLS and hypnosis is still unknown. However, it is believed that you reach a state of complete relaxation which relieves you and allows you to sleep better at nights.

These alternate treatment methods of RLS have not been evaluated with any clinical trials. All the data available only gives us possible relationships between these treatment methods and the condition. However, there are several anecdotal evidences available to encourage individuals suffering from RLS to try these simple and safe methods out. Today, new techniques like aroma therapy are also being used. The common thing between all these treatment methods is that they all focus on relaxing the body. When your body is completely relaxed, you can fall asleep easily and also be free from the painful and distressing symptoms of RLS.

Homeopathy

There are several effective remedies recommended by homeopathic doctors. Some of these remedies are not instant but they can give your great relief with consistency. The first remedy that is usually recommended is Causticum. You must consume them at a 12C dilution to relieve RLS symptoms. You can also try Tarentula hispanica at 12 C dilution thrice each day. You must continue these medicines till you see any improvement in the symptoms.

6. Lifestyle Changes to Reduce RLS

The lifestyle that you lead may not be helping you manage your RLS symptoms. There are instances when these symptoms are actually aggravated by your habits. Sometimes, were are not even aware that a simple habit like drinking coffee can be the cause for those painful night awakenings and the relentless need to wake up every night. In fact, when I was asked to make a couple of lifestyle changes it almost seemed like an "aha" moment for me. The symptoms were reduced considerably and I was also able to function a lot better.

a. Managing Stress

If you are stressed or anxious, your RLS symptoms will aggravate. Before you make any other lifestyle change, you must make sure that you find ways to stat stress free for better results.

Managing stress will also improve the response that you have to traditional RLS treatment. Here are some tips that you can follow to keep yourself free from stress at all times:

- Breathe Deeply: This technique works very well when you experience RLS symptoms after a long tiring day. When you breathe in deeply, your body gets a sudden boost of oxygen. This is useful not only in refreshing your mind completely, but will also reduce tightness in your muscles that is caused from a lack of oxygen. When your muscles do not get enough oxygen, they tend to cramp up or become extremely hard and tight. This is one of the primary causes of the tingling and painful sensations that your experience in your legs when you have RLS. When my symptoms become very severe I spend several minutes breathing deeply.

This not only reduces the symptoms but also helps me sleep better when the symptoms calm down. I have noticed that breathing is a technique that is used in most relaxation techniques. Whether it is yoga or even working out at the gym, breathing is a very integral part of it. Whenever you feel like a bundle of nerves, just breathe in and breathe out. Make sure you breathe in through your nose and breathe out through your mouth. To make sure that you are breathing correctly, place your hands at the sides of your ribs. When you breathe in, there should be a sideward movement of your hands. That is when you know that your rib cage is working and expanding. This technique of breathing is most useful. If you practice yoga, you will be introduced to several other breathing techniques. Pick one that works best for you and your RLS symptoms can be managed quite easily.

- Mindfulness Meditation: This technique works really well if you are having trouble sleeping. When you are too stressed out, you will find it hard to sleep even if you do not have a condition like RLS. The primary reason for this type of sleep deprivation is the inability to let go of troubling thoughts. We tend to ponder over the uneventful things that occurred. When you maintain a sleep diary, you will be able to address any source of distress a lot better.

Mindfulness Meditation is a great way to keep yourself focused and free from stress. The main goal of this type of meditation is to be mindful of the present. You must pay attention only to your present moment and detach yourself from negative thoughts. The idea is to allow these thoughts to occur as they do without really judging them. So, you are free from any stress caused by these negative thoughts.

To practice this method, find a quiet place in your home. Do not push yourself to meditate for several minutes in the beginning. Start with a goal of about 5 minutes initially. Shift your focus to your breath. Inhale and exhale consistently and focus on this entirely. You can either meditate in the morning or in the evening. When you have RLS symptoms, meditating just before going to bed can have a great influence on your symptoms and on your ability to sleep better.

Mindfulness meditation also has a calming effect on your nervous system and your muscles. This reduces cramps and painful sensations that are common when you are suffering from RLS. When the nervous system is fully calmed down, the neurotransmitters like dopamine are also regulated well. This makes sure that the symptoms of RLS are reduced. Any anxiety that might be triggering your RLS symptoms is controlled when you practice Mindfulness Meditation on a regular basis.

- **Exercise:** Exercise works very well on your stress and anxiety. However, when you have RLS symptoms, you must make sure that you do not indulge in extremely strenuous work outs as they aggravate the symptoms. Mild exercises that help you relax the muscles are ideal to relieve you from your RLS symptoms as well as anxiety. When you have a routine for your workout, you will see that the stress you experience is also highly reduced.

When you exercise, a hormone called endorphin is released. This hormone is commonly called the happy hormone and is vital for reducing stress. This is one of the primary reasons why you feel completely refreshed after a good workout. Next, your muscles are completely relaxed when you work out. This can help reduce the cramps and the sensations that you experience in your legs or in other part s of your body when you have RLS.

- Avoid Overworking yourself: For most people, biggest source of stress is their work. For some of them, it is because they are not happy with the job that they are currently in. For others, it is the tendency to overwork that makes them more prone to stress and anxiety. If you have RLS, you must ensure that you do not work just before you go to bed. Working from your bed on a laptop, can be the worst thing that you do when you already have RLS. If you have stressful thoughts of your work just before going to bed, you will not be able to fall asleep. In addition to that, your RLS symptoms will also act up, making night awakenings more.

If you can calm your mind down with any activity that helps you, you must make it a habit. For some, a cup of warm tea or milk works. For others, reading does the trick. If you like to practice any other form of relaxation like inhaling essential oils or taking a bath, it would be a good idea to make sure you do it when your day has been hard and stressful.

b. Drink Lots of Water

Staying hydrated could be the answer to the distress caused by RLS. Dehydration due to reduced water consumption could lead to severe symptoms as the muscles tend to cramp up in the absence of water. If you have observed athletes, they tend to drink a lot of water when they are working out. Some of them may also use electrolytes. This prevents cramps in the muscles due to dehydration. When you are dehydrated, you also feel more exhausted throughout the day. This leads to stress which, in turn leads to RLS symptoms.

Our body requires close to 80 minerals as I mentioned before. You also need adequate vitamins in order to feel relieved of the symptoms of RLS. However, when your body does not have enough water, most of these minerals and nutrients are not dissolved properly. So, they are of no use to the body at all. Also, you need enough water for these nutrients to be transported to various parts of your body. Studies have also revealed that drinking enough water boosts the performance of your brain as well.

Most websites would recommend that you drink 8 glasses of water every day. However, what works best is to drink water whenever you feel thirsty and after your meals. If you do not have the habit of drinking water at all, you may keep a target for each day and drink water accordingly.

c. Reduce Caffeine Consumption

As mentioned before, Caffeine is one of the triggers for RLS symptoms. Caffeine also reduces your ability to fall asleep. You must avoid caffeine as it is also a diuretic. This means that coffee can dehydrate you causing cramps and other common RLS symptoms.

If you are used to drinking coffee, try to replace it with another beverage such as green tea that is beneficial in treating your RLS symptoms. You may also try a special tea like chamomile tea that is not only refreshing but also completely relaxing.

Remember, the coffee is not the only source of caffeine. Aerated drinks, energy drinks and several confectionaries contain coffee. So, make sure you check the ingredients of all the products that you consume.

Caffeine also interferes with the reaction of the medication that you are taking for your RLS symptoms. It prevents the cells from absorbing the medication that you take, thereby rendering the useless!

d. Reduce Alcohol Consumption

Alcohol consumption should be stopped entirely when you have RLS symptoms. If you have severe, symptoms, especially, you must cut this out entirely. Most individuals who have sleep related disorders believe that alcohol can help them fall asleep. This is a common myth that simply aggravates all the symptoms of RLS.

Alcohol should particularly be avoided when you are just going to bed. Remember that alcohol is a dehydrating agent. So, consuming alcohol results in leg cramps and painful sensations when you are trying to fall asleep. Even periodic leg movements increase with the consumption of alcohol.

For those who are used to consuming alcohol, there could be RLS symptoms as a result of the withdrawals experienced when you try to reduce the amount of alcohol consumed. When you experience this, make sure that you consult your healthcare provider for options to manage these aggravated symptoms. You may also try relaxation techniques such as yoga, tai chi, breathing exercise, and hot beverages before you go to bed.

e. Make Ergonomic Changes

Ergonomic changes mean making changes in your posture whenever you are working and also throughout your day. If you are sitting in a rather uncomfortable position all day, there are chances that your cramps will increase when you go to bed. This can be relieved by either performing simple exercises when you are at work, walking around and also changing your position regularly.

According to testimonies of RLS patients, using a stool that is high is a great way to improve your posture. When you are seated in this manner, your legs are left dangling. This will improve the blood circulation to your legs. You also have more mobility, allowing you to exercise your legs and move them around to prevent them from cramping.

You may also have to make changes in the way you travel. For many individuals, the symptoms aggravate and become very intense when they are travelling by air. This is because the space available is very small. You may also have to stay in the same place and in the same position for several hours. This can be avoided when you opt for an aisle seat when you are travelling by air. This prevents any disturbance to your co passengers. You can also stretch your legs or even walk around for a while when you begin to experience these symptoms.

Lastly, improve your posture when you sleep. This is made possible when you have the right mattress to sleep on. Make sure your mattress does not sink in too deep, making your movement restricted. These lifestyle changes have brought significant relief to most individuals who experience RLS symptoms. I can also vouch for these lifestyle changes as I have seen that they also help me carry out my activities throughout the day more peacefully.

f. Reduce Sugar Consumption

Sugar is another common trigger for RLS. When you increase your sugar consumption, the symptoms tend to increase. One possible reason for this is that sugar reduces your magnesium absorption. You know the importance of magnesium in controlling the symptoms of RLS. Try to avoid sugar in your diet. You must make sure that you do not consume foods that contain too many preservatives. Another important advice is that "sugar free" tablets that are used as a replacement for sugar must also be avoided. They have the same effect as sugar and may be more harmful as they are artificial products. Another important lifestyle change that you need to make is including exercises to ease the symptoms. However, the exercises that you practice when you have RLS symptoms are quite different. The next chapter deals with this subject in greater detail.

g. Changes to Make in Your Diet

The food that you eat plays a very important role in your RLS symptoms. We have already discussed about the nutrients that are necessary to avoid RLS symptoms. In fact, there are certain nutrient deficiencies that have been listed as the causal factors of RLS. Making dietary changes has proved useful for many friends who suffer from RLS. If you visit the online blogs for RLS, you will see that changing the diet is listed as one of the main natural remedies for this syndrome. There are a few foods that should be included in your diet to prevent RLS symptoms or to improve the condition.

Foods Rich in Iron

Along with iron supplementation, eating foods that are high in iron is one of the most reliable ways of replenishing the iron content in your body. Since RLS symptoms are caused by iron deficiency, this is one of the most important inclusions that you need to make in your diet. According to the National Institute of Health, when there is an iron deficiency in the body, neurological symptoms are common. It may also lead to a compromised immune system along with poor cognitive abilities.

The best sources of iron are animal proteins such as fish, poultry and read meat. There are several options for vegetarians as well. You can consume lentils, pinto, soy, navy, kidney beans and also black beans for a high iron source. You can also include green leafy vegetables, asparagus and green peas in your diet.

Foods containing Magnesium

Magnesium, in several forms is considered to be one of the best treatment options for individuals with RLS. The University of Maryland Medical Centre has stated that including magnesium in your diet can relieve RLS. Another study published in the August 2009 edition of "Sleep" by the Department of Psychotherapy at the Albert Ludwig's University also confirms this.

The throbbing sensations are reduced and sleep is also improved when you consume at least 250 mg of magnesium every day. Even the urge to wake up and move is reduced when you consume magnesium. The best sources of magnesium are spinach, nuts, legumes, whole grains and seeds. Basically foods that are high in fibres are also great sources of magnesium. Consuming organically grown foods in magnesium rich soil is a better option and is a higher source of the mineral.

Foods Containing Folate

A folate is a form of Vitamin B that is soluble in water. This is a very important component for the production of new cells in the body. Folates are necessary in replenishing the RBC levels in the body. This can prevent anemia and can help prevent the symptoms of RLS. Any food that contains folates or folic acid is extremely beneficial in relieving your RLS symptoms. According to a study published by the Canadian Medical Association Journal, it was observed that patients who suffered from RLS saw relief from symptoms by consuming just about 10 mg of folic acid every day. So, make sure that this food group is a major part of your diet.

The foods that are rich in folates are beef liver, spinach, beans, broccoli, green peas, fortified grains and fortified cereal and pasta.

When it comes to nutrition, you must be prepared for one thing. Do not expect to see the changes immediately. Of course, you may find temporary relief. But, our body takes some time to replenish your nutrients. Whether it is the manifestation of a deficiency related disease or whether it is recovery from a deficiency related disease you need at least 4 weeks to see any symptom or improvement respectively.

You see nutrition only helps us make our body better by building it up gradually. Even the blood cells that we have last for a maximum of 120 days. What this means is that in a period of three months our entire blood is renewed. Every six months the proteins in the body are all replaced. Even the ones in our DNA, apparently! Now if you are wondering what I am trying to say here, it is pretty simple. Consistency is the key to benefiting from your diet.

You see, even when you have a deficiency, it is quite unlikely that you will notice any symptoms for at least 4 weeks. Even if you remove a certain nutrient from your diet completely, your body has enough reserves to last for an entire month! It is only when the cells are replaced that the disease ravages the body.

Our body functions just like a plant that has not been watered for ages. Imagine you just start watering a plant that has wilted completely. There is a chance that the leaves may look healthy and perked up for a bit. However, the plant will look healthy only when the old and dry leaves fall off. Just like you have to wait for the old leaves to fall off, you also have to wait for your old cells to be replaced entirely. All you can do is feed your body well and wait patiently for the results to show.

When we have the right nutrients, the entire physiology of the body changes and it returns to a balanced state. Your health will see a holistic improvement only when you make sure that the body has all the nutrients that it needs to function properly.

Chapter 9: RLS as a Withdrawal Symptom

When you are a habitual consumer of alcohol or opiates, there are severe withdrawal symptoms. RLS is a common withdrawal symptoms that is experienced especially when a person is withdrawing from opiates. The symptoms are usually severe and may even occur with the same intensity during the day. This prevents an individual from functioning properly. It is also very hard to prescribe any medication to provide relief from RLS symptoms during withdrawals. There are only a few medications that are recommended including:

- Clondine: This medicine is used to reduce agitation, aches in the muscles, cramping and even a runny nose.

- Benzodiazepines: These medicines induce sleep and allow one to get immediate relief from the symptoms. However, this is a very strong medicine which should not be consumed for more than 5 days when you are feeling withdrawal symptoms.

- Baclofen: This is only a temporary medicine that is given for an individual who is suffering from opiate related RLS symptoms. However, there isn't enough evidence to prove that this medicine is efficient. So, it is not recommended often despite being one of the few medicines that are available for RLS during withdrawal symptoms.

Withdrawal symptoms are not life threatening. However, any wrong medication may cause adverse effects. The frequency of all the withdrawal symptoms could increase when strong medicines are prescribed. So, non-medicinal treatments are best recommended when you are trying to manage opiate related RLS symptoms. Here are certain methods that have been useful for many people who are managing both these conditions:

140

Hot and Cold Treatment: Alternating between hot and cold treatment will relieve the cramps almost instantly. This treatment is particularly useful when you are withdrawing from opiates as this is a relaxing procedure. You can also feel relief from cramping in other parts of the body, mostly the abdomen. You may either wash your legs with hot and cold water, directing strong spurts of water on your calves. It is also a good idea to alternate between a hot pack and an ice pack when you are going to bed.

Weighing Down Your Legs: This method is used to actually "smother" the legs to prevent your RLS symptoms. Using a heavy blanket and wrapping it around your legs is known to prevent the symptoms of RLS. You can also add small weights on your blanket in order to stop the movements of your legs. This works very well when you are experiencing violent movements of your legs due to opiate related RLS. You can even place a heavy pillow on your legs in order to stop term from moving so severely. This is most useful when you have periodic limb movements along with RLS.

Lying Down on Your Stomach: Changing your sleeping position is a great way to sleep better. When you are withdrawing from opiates, you will experience several other symptoms including nausea, dizziness and abdominal cramps in addition to RLS. You can get rid of all these problems by sleeping on your stomach. Lie in this position for at least half an hour. You must make sure that the mattress that you lie on is hard. If it sinks in, you will not experience any relief from the symptoms. Lying down on the floor is the best option. If you have a tiled floor that might be cooler, you will definitely see immediate results.

Stretching: A couple of stretches have been mentioned in the previous chapter. You can try them out in order to find some relief from your RLS symptoms. Do not over stretch. You can stretch your muscles every time you feel the symptoms. Even slightly rubbing down on your legs when the symptoms start will relieve you from the symptoms. Stretching relaxes the muscles and reduces cramping. Periodic movements also reduce if you stretch regularly. These exercises are also extremely relaxing and will allow you to sleep better as well.

Compression Socks: This is recommended when your symptoms are too severe. For many people with opiate withdrawals, fatigue is a common. You need some method to cope with the condition that does not require any effort from your end. Compression clothing is the best option for individuals who are experiencing multiple withdrawal symptoms. These "socks" clench your muscles almost as if they are massaging them. This allows you to sleep without any spasms or painful sensations. The need to move your legs around also reduces when you have RLS symptoms also reduce when you use compression socks.

Wrapping your Legs: This works like compression clothes. However, wrapping your legs with a tension bandage is not so tightly fitted. This is recommended when numbness is a primary symptom that you experience. You also need to ensure that blood circulation is higher in your legs when you feel numbness. This serves a dual purpose of relieving your legs from the RLS symptoms while keeping your blood circulation intact. You can wrap your legs immediately after a hot and cold treatment for best results. Some people also like to wrap their legs with a bar of soap. It is believed that this can alleviate the RLS symptoms to a greater extent.

There are several support groups available to help you cope with opiate or alcohol related withdrawals. These groups help you cope with the emotional trauma caused by substance abuse. These psychological issues are amplified due to sleeplessness.

You can also seek the assistance of an authorised sleep clinic. There are specialised techniques that will help you relax and sleep better. If you are already seeing a therapist to help you cope with addiction, make sure you tell him or her about the RLS symptoms that you are experiencing. Self-medication is never recommended as it may have fatal consequences. You must also improve your diet and your lifestyle when you are dealing with the double threat of RLS symptoms and opiate withdrawals. This will strengthen your body and make it able to respond to all the treatment methods employed.

Chapter 10: How to Improve Sleep

You can improve your sleep pattern even when you have RLS. For most people, including me, the idea of sleeping peacefully seems quite distant. But, I realised that there are some good sleeping habits that can improve the quality of your sleep. When you follow a few simple tips, you should also be able to reduce the night time awakenings.

Sleep habits are very easy to cultivate. They require a few simple changes in the sleep timing and your sleeping patterns. Good and healthy sleeping patterns are also known as sleep hygiene. Here are some sleep practices that you can follow consistently for better sleep.

Follow a routine: There is a fixed pattern to our sleep. We always feel sleepy at a certain time of the day and are able to work and perform activities. You also have a fixed number of hours that you can stay asleep. This is called a circadian rhythm. In common terms, it is called a body clock. You see, our body loves a routine. When you maintain one, you will be able to keep up with this sleep pattern too. So, it is a good idea to have a particular time for going to bed. Also, make sure you sleep in the same room and on the same bed every night. This brings a sense of familiarity that allows your mind to relax as well.

Find one relaxation technique: Make it a point to find a good relaxation technique that works for you. There are different techniques like smelling essential oils, lighting scented candles, meditating etc. that you can choose from. Even with this technique, maintain consistency. Your body should be familiar with the relaxation method that you follow. So, whenever you start your relaxation routine, it is a trigger for your body to fall asleep. Your body responds to some cues and releases the necessary hormones that are meant to induce sleep.

144

Do not nap in the afternoon: Many successful businessmen swear by power naps in the afternoon. These naps, no doubt, help them improve their performance. However, their quality of sleep at night is highly compromised. Especially when you have a sleeping condition like RLS, a nap must be avoided. This will make you more restless towards the evening. You can find other methods to relax when you are at work. Instead of sleeping, you can read a book, listen to music or even take a walk. Getting some fresh air when I feel drowsy and lethargic at the office works best for me. Find an alternative to sleep and you will notice better quality of sleep at night.

Make sure you exercise: When you have RLS, it is impossible to tire yourself with a vigorous workout and then fall asleep. This is because heavy workout tends to aggravate your RLS symptoms. However, when you have no physical activity at all, it does take a toll on your body. Metabolism is slower and you feel lazy. However, the fact that you have so much energy left in your body will not even help you sleep. So, try some light work outs through the day. Just before you go to bed, stretch your legs out to sleep better.

Check your sleep environment: The room that you are sleeping in should be evaluated thoroughly. The temperature should be maintained at about 60 degrees. If your room is noisy or is facing a street that is noisy, you may not be able to stay sleep. In such cases, using a thick curtain or even closing your window can help you sleep better. Avoid distractions like televisions in the room that you are going to sleep in. Lastly, avoid any light in the room. If there is a street light that falls into your room, sleep might be disturbed. There are many options like ear plugs, eye shades, blackout curtains, air conditioners, humidifiers etc. that you can use to improve your sleep environment.

Use better mattresses and pillows: Your mattress should be comfortable and should offer enough support. If you have been using the same mattress for over 8 years, then you may need to change it for better sleep. You see even mattresses and pillows have a certain life expectancy. When you change your mattresses, also put in some effort to make your bed look nice. Use better sheets and pillowcases. When you make your room more inviting for sleep you will sleep better. Just make sure that the fabrics that you use do not have allergens. Also avoid any objects that may make you slip or even fall. If you have the problem of night awakenings, the last thing you want in an injury.

Watch what you eat and drink: Just before you fall asleep, make sure you do not consume any alcohol. Avoid cigarettes before you fall asleep. Some people also have the habit of eating a really heavy meal before they sleep. This can actually disrupt your sleep. If the food that you have eaten is very spicy, you may have indigestion or discomfort when you try to sleep. Also, try to eat at least 2 hours before you fall asleep. When your stomach is light, you are more relaxed. You will also notice that your sleep quality becomes a lot better.

Make sure you wind down: The body needs to calm down and shift to a sleep mode. If you keep it engaged and working to the last minute, you might find it harder to sleep. Take all the sleeping material out of your room. Using laptops and other electronic devices is definitely not recommended. The light that these devices emanate activates parts of your brain making it difficult for you to fall asleep. Make sure you use the last one hour before you sleep to do something that is calming. Reading is an age old practice that has always helped people fall asleep.

Try a different room till you feel tired: In case you need to work before you sleep, allot a different room for this. Your bed must be used only for sleeping. This helps your mind strengthen the sleep and bed association. This is another type of cue that your brain uses in order to help you sleep better. On the other hand, if you tend to do stressful things like your business reports etc. while you are on your bed or in your bed room, your body and mind associates this space with anxiety. So, you find it harder to fall asleep.

Change the lights in your room: Like I mentioned before, the body follows a certain rhythm that is triggered by certain cues. Light is one of the most important cues for the circadian rhythm of our body. If you have very bright lights in your room during the evenings, your body will not respond correctly. For our body, it is still too bright for it to shut down. So, the melatonin levels will remain low, not letting you fall asleep. It is a good idea to use dim lights, preferably lampshades in the room that you are going to sleep in. You may also turn the lights down just before you go to bed.

If none of these methods work, you may need to speak to a sleep professional. Maintain a sleep diary as part of your sleep hygiene. When you follow these patterns regularly, even your RLS symptoms will reduce considerably.

Whilst I am talking about improving sleep, I have improved my sleep dramatically with the three remedies listed below. I do realise I have already said this under the treatment section of this book but I am repeating what works for me again, as it also fits into this chapter about improving sleep.

a) I do stretch exercises first - see remedy number 55.

b) Then I massage my feet and calves with Glysolid cream - remedy number 4.

c) Then I push my legs against sand bags - remedy number 7.

When I sometimes wake up during the night, with RLS, I repeat these 3 methods again (a,b,c) and it usually works and I fall asleep again almost immediately.

Chapter 11: Why is Sleep Deprivation Dangerous?

RLS is not restricted to the physical symptoms that you experience. That is why; this condition can actually interfere in your life as well. In the introduction to this book I mentioned how the RLS symptoms devastated the personal life of women who suffered from this condition. You see, sleep deprivation is the biggest concern with RLS. While it may not seem like that big a deal, when you are unable to sleep for days on end, it does drive you up the wall. Believe me, I know! I am a business woman with a large to-do list, at all times. I have to be laser focused in everything that I do in business. One can't be laser focused when one hasn't had a good night sleep for 2 weeks. That was me, before I started investigating RLS seriously. I knew things would have to change and I WAS going to solve my RLS and get some good night sleep once again. I have suffered from sleep deprivation for many years!

Sleep deprivation is not limited to fatigue and stress. This can lead to several emotional problems as well. In fact, research shows that sleep deprivation can be life threatening. Therefore, RLS symptoms should be addressed as early as possible to avoid any untoward consequences from sleep deprivation. There are several things that can go wrong when you do not have enough sleep. Testimonies from people with RLS have revealed that people develop habits like gambling in order to cope with the inability to sleep. I have spoken to several peers to understand what effect sleep deprivation has had on them. Listed below are the common observations:

1. How the Body is Affected

Sleep is one of the primary requirements of the body. This is just as important as eating or even breathing. When you fall asleep, the body is at work taking care of our physical and mental health. This helps prepare you for all the activities that you have in store for the next day.

In case of children, growth spurts occur when they are sleeping. This is true even in case of adolescents. It is when they are asleep that the growth hormone is released. These hormones are very important in building your muscles. When you sleep, all the damaged cells and tissues are repaired. The onset of puberty is also determined by sleep. That is why, adolescent girls who do not sleep enough notice problems in their menstrual cycles.

When you are sleep deprived, your body perceives this as a threat. As a result, it goes into a defensive mode. You will see that the function is impaired and even your cognitive abilities are weakened when you are unable to sleep. Your body will give you signs in the form of excessive yawning and also too much sleepiness when you are sleep deprived. When these initial symptoms are ignored, the body also shuts off your decision making abilities. Your ability to take decisions and stay alert prevents you from falling asleep when you are performing an activity like driving. However, when you are sleep deprived, you may fall asleep while carrying out high risk activities leading to injuries. You cannot even use stimulants like caffeine to override your body's need to sleep.

The effects of substances like alcohol are also magnified when you are unable to fall asleep. According to a research conducted by the Harvard Medical School, sleeping for less than five hours every night can increase the risk of death from accidents by 15%. The quality of life is lowered considerably when you do not sleep enough.

2. How the Nervous System is Affected

All the information that you have and all the information that you receive from the world around you is processed by your highly efficient central nervous system. Even this information highway requires enough sleep in order to function normally. When you are sleeping, your brain is resting but is not entirely inactive. All your neurons are being repaired and replaced to create new pathways to process the information. This repair is possible only when you are sleeping as the proteins necessary for cell repair are released when you are asleep.

When you are sleep deprived, these pathways are highly compromised. So, you are unable to concentrate on your activities. In addition to that, you will not be able to learn anything new either as your ability to process any new information is reduced. Memory is affected as the information is not retained either. This effect is seen in both your long term and your short term memory. Creativity becomes close to nil when you are sleep deprived. You are also unable to make proper decisions when you are sleep deprived. The emotions that you experience are intense. This leads to mood swings and even agitation. On the whole, all your cognitive abilities become impaired when you are sleep deprived.

If deprivation of sleep is prolonged, the effects are intensified as well. You are prone to hallucinations. Any sleeping condition like narcolepsy is also magnified. For those who experience mania or manic depression, sleep deprivation acts as a very important trigger. The other risks associated with sleep deprivation are suicidal thoughts, paranoia, depression and impulsive behaviour. This may lead to actions that can cause harm or even lead to fatalities.

The nervous system triggers off certain defence mechanism to cope with sleep deprivation. It attempts to make up for the lack of sleep by setting of certain mechanisms. One such mechanism is known as micro sleep. You tend to doze off for just a few minutes without even realising this. Sometimes, micro sleep can be as short as a few seconds. However, it is extremely risky when you are driving or when you handle heavy machines at your work place. You become a lot more prone to accidents due to micro sleep. The National, Heart, Lung and Blood Institute has reported several tragic accidents that involved ships, air planes and even nuclear reactors. All these accidents were the result of sleep deprivation in the person who was operating these machines.

3. How Immunity is Affected

The immune system is active when you are sleeping. This is when all the protective mechanisms in the body are initiated. Infections are fought with the help of antibodies. The immune system also produces cytokines which are used to kill bacteria, viruses and other germs that have infected the body. These substances are also helpful in putting you to sleep. When your body is rejuvenated due to sleep, the immune system is strengthened to defend you against the illnesses. When you are sleep deprived, the immune system does not have an opportunity to rejuvenate. The Mayo Clinic reported that most people who have trouble with their immune system are often sleep deprived. When you don't sleep enough, the time taken to recover from illnesses also increases. You are at the risk of developing diseases like diabetes when you have had prolonged sleep deprivation.

4. How Your Breathing is Affected

The primary cause for respiratory issues when you are sleep deprived is a weakened immune system. You are more prone to developing flu and other breathing problems. For those who already have chronic lung problems, treatment is ineffective when they are sleep deprived. It is also possible that you develop chronic respiratory problems as a result of sleep deprivation.

6. How Your Digestive System is Affected

If you are reading this book, you are probably familiar with the effects of sleep deprivation on your digestive system. This seems to be the first part that is affected. Bowel movement is disrupted causing extreme uneasiness. You also do not feel like eating very often. In fact, you are so tired sometimes that you just do not want to put in any efforts to even eat. This is feeling that I lived with for several years. Even exercising and medication does not help you fall asleep as your body believes that you have eaten enough. Yes, this is true. Whenever you do not sleep well, a hormone called cortisol is released. This is a stress hormone. Also, the level of another hormone called leptin drops drastically. This imbalance in the hormone levels tells your body that you have eaten enough. But sometimes, the effect is quite contrary.

In some cases, instead of the hormones mentioned above, a third biochemical agent called gherlin comes into play. This is an appetite stimulant. So, you feel the need to binge uncontrollably. Another effect is that insulin levels become higher when you tend to binge. This is a very serious effect on the body as the combination of gherlin and insulin increases the storage of fat in your body. This not only increases the chance of developing diabetes type 2, a possible causal factor for RLS, but also makes your obese or overweight.

7. How Your Cardiovascular System is Affected

If you gain weight as a result of sleep deprivation, the immediate effect is seen on your cardiovascular system. Weight gain is almost equivalent to problems with the heart. You need to have enough sleep in order for your body to heal the blood vessels in the heart. Sometimes, due to stress or exertion, these blood vessels could get damaged. However, if you are sleep deprived, you will develop chronic health problems like strokes and high blood pressure. A study conducted by the Harvard Medical School on individuals with hypertension showed that the blood pressure remained elevated despite medication in individuals who were deprived of sleep for even one night.

With all these risks to various parts of your body, getting enough sleep is vital. So, even when you notice the slightest chances of a sleep disorder, visit your doctor immediately. Most often, it is the lack of sleep, rather than the condition itself that causes serious problems.

Chapter 12: If Your Partner has RLS

In many cases, it is the spouse or the partner who brings the condition to the notice of an expert. If a person has only periodic limb movements that have not extended into Restless Leg Syndrome, he may not even be aware of the fact that his limbs move uncontrollably after he has fallen asleep.

Being the partner of someone who has sleep issues is not easy. If you are reading this book to understand the problem that your partner is facing, let me tell you that you play a vital role in his or her recovery. Yes, if you can work along with your partner to ease this condition, the results are faster. You will also not have to face the problem of sleep disturbances when you can help your partner overcome these symptoms. When you work together, you can avert several issues that are caused within a relationship as a result of RLS.

Studies conducted by the Florida Sleep Institute have shown that close to 80% of individuals with RLS combined with periodic limb movements face distress in their relationship. There is enough evidence to suggest that the person who has RLS can trigger insomnia in his partner. However, doctors suggest that a couple should make an effective treatment plan that will help both of them cope with the condition.

First, help your partner relax if he or she experiences RLS. Massaging the legs is one of the best solutions to ease the Restless leg syndrome. When you make a pact to massage your partner's legs be aware of your threshold for assistance. While it may seem ok once in a while, it could become too tedious after some time. You can also look for other means of relaxation.

Take some time off with each other every day. You can take a walk down the street. Just make sure that your walk is relaxed and not very vigorous as it may trigger the RLS symptoms making it unbearable for you. In addition to this, sudden exertion just before you sleep can really mess with your biological clock. You could read a book, sip some tea or even pursue relaxation techniques like meditation together. This not only benefits the person with RLS but can help you as well.

In case the symptoms do occur anyway, apply some pressure on your partner's legs. You could place your legs over your partner's legs and wait for the symptoms to calm down. For many people sitting on their partner's leg for a while helps ease the symptoms. You could even use a heavy blanket and drape it around your partner's legs for immediate relief.

If the symptoms are too severe, you may also consider using separate blankets. This will help you sleep better and prevent irritation and anger within a relationship. You may place a bar of soap under your partner's blanket as it is believed to be of great assistance in relieving RLS symptoms.

Do not lose your intimacy. This is one of the main reasons for the issues within a relationship. Include sex as a part of your RLS treatment program. This is one of the many ways to alleviate the symptoms as well. It has been proved through studies that RLS symptoms can be reduced after an orgasm. Although there is no definite reason for this, it helps. Of course, you will also be able maintain emotional security within your relationship when you are intimate with your partner.

Remember to be supportive. Your partner will have to give up habits like alcohol, caffeine etc. which can be extremely difficult. This may also result in a lot of irritability in your partner. You need to be prepared for that. Encourage your partner to get rid of these habits. You need to help him or her abstain by providing some form of distraction. IF you can think of simple activities to do together, you should be able to get rid of any tension in the relationship. Try to keep your partner's mind stimulated. This is also known to help reduce the symptoms of RLS as certain sections of the brain are activated.

If none of these methods work, you can also seek couples therapy. You need to be a little understanding towards the condition. As you have already read until now, this is a condition that is beyond the control of your partner. However, when you work as a team, you can most certainly overcome this together.

Conclusion

There is a lot of on-going research in order to find new cures for Restless Leg Syndrome. The results of these studies are a great source of hope for people who are dealing with severe symptoms.

One of the first devices to deal with RLS was approved by the FDA in the month of June in 2014. This is a pad called Relaxis. You can lie in bed and place the pad on your legs or on the affected part of your body. The vibrations in this device magnify and then stop, acting like an alternative to actually getting up and moving. This device is highly recommended for individuals who are taking medicines for relief from RLS. This device will be available on prescription very soon in the United States of America.

According to a recent study, a medicine called pregablin has outperformed the standard medicines used in RLS treatment. According to Richard Allen from the John Hopkins University School of Medicine, this medicine works just as well as Pramipexole which is commonly suggested for individuals with RLS. However, there is an added advantage to this new medicine. Many people find that their symptoms become worse with the use of Pramipexole. However, pregablin has no such negative effects.

There are several on-going tests to see how effective this new medication is. These tests are dedicated to understanding how effective the new medication will be in improving the quality of life along with the quality of life.

There are many gaps in our understanding of this common condition. However, today, we are a lot more aware of the causes and treatment of this condition than we were a few decades ago. There are several tests that are being conducted to find the ideal medicine to cure this condition. Recent studies and results suggest that we are very much on that progressive path. In the meanwhile, we must remember that RLS is a progressive condition. The sooner we deal with it and make necessary changes, the better our lives will be.

Thank you for reading this book. I hope that you found it as informative as it was intended to be. The idea of this book was to equip you with practical steps to deal with this condition. I hope that it has met that requirement. I wish you all a long and healthy life free from the severe symptoms or RLS.

Some remedies worked for me, so they might work for you! Don't hesitate and start trying one of them TONIGHT! I truly hope that you will find a remedy that works for you!

Good luck!

Emily - ex RLS sufferer.

Well, that's not true, I am not an ex-sufferer. I am still a RLS sufferer but I apply remedies to make my symptoms do-able and I **do** get lots of good nights sleep, which I couldn't say 5 years ago!

Published by IMB Publishing 2015

Copyright and Trademarks: This publication is Copyrighted 2015 by IMB Publishing. All products, publications, software and services mentioned and recommended in this publication are protected by trademarks. In such instance, all trademarks & copyright belong to the respective owners. All rights reserved. No part of this book may be reproduced or transferred in any form or by any means, graphic, electronic, or mechanical, including photocopying, recording, taping, or by any information storage retrieval system, without the written permission of the authors. Pictures used in this book are either royalty free pictures bought from stock-photo websites or have the source mentioned underneath the picture.

Disclaimer and Legal Notice: This product is not legal or medical advice and should not be interpreted in that manner. You need to do your own due-diligence to determine if the content of this product is right for you. The authors and the affiliates of this product are not liable for any damages or losses associated with the content in this product. While every attempt has been made to verify the information shared in this publication, neither the author nor the affiliates assume any responsibility for errors, omissions or contrary interpretation of the subject matter herein. Any perceived slights to any specific person(s) or organization(s) are purely unintentional. We have no control over the nature, content and availability of the web sites listed in this book.

The inclusion of any web site links does not necessarily imply a recommendation or endorse the views expressed within them. IMB Publishing takes no responsibility for, and will not be liable for, the websites being temporarily unavailable or being removed from the Internet.

The accuracy and completeness of information provided herein and opinions stated herein are not guaranteed or warranted to produce any particular results, and the advice and strategies, contained herein may not be suitable for every individual. The author shall not be liable for any loss incurred as a consequence of the use and application, directly or indirectly, of any information presented in this work. This publication is designed to provide information in regard to the subject matter covered.

The information included in this book has been compiled to give an overview of the subject and detail some of the symptoms, treatments etc. that are available. It is not intended to give medical advice. For a firm diagnosis of any health condition, and for a treatment plan suitable for you and your dog, you should consult your veterinarian or consultant.

The writer of this book and the publisher are not responsible for any damages or negative consequences following any of the treatments or methods highlighted in this book. Website links are for informational purposes and should not be seen as a personal endorsement; the same applies to the products detailed in this book. The reader should also be aware that although the web links included were correct at the time of writing, they may become out of date in the future.

18353956R00092

Made in the USA
Middletown, DE
03 March 2015